Proven Herbal Blends

A Rational Approach to Prevention and Remedy

Condensed from *The Scientific Validation of Herbal Medicine*

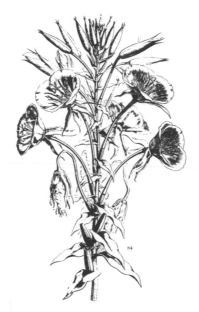

Daniel B. Mowrey, Ph.D.

Keats Publishing, Inc. New Canaan, Connecticut

PROVEN HERBAL BLENDS
Copyright © 1986 by Cormorant Books
Published by arrangement with the author
All Rights Reserved

No part of this book may be reproduced in any form without the written consent of the publisher

Printed in the United States of America

Published by Keats Publishing, Inc.
27 Pine Street (Box 876)
New Canaan, Connecticut 06840

Table of Contents

PREFACE

This book, like the one from which it is condensed—**The Scientific Validation of Herbal Medicine**—seeks to educate people on the rational use of herbs and herbal blends. You will not find much in the way of folk medicine here. Or mythology. Or plagarism (one of the real problems in herbalism). The quality of this work rests squarely on the author's ability to evaluate the reliability and validity of source material, be it scientific publications, clinical data or ethnopharmacological information. Being a condensation, this work must abbreviate wherever possible and yet still retain the flavor of the original, a task which has proven arduous and frustrating.

Every chapter and every section of **The Scientific Validation of Herbal Medicine** is retained in this book, but in a shorter version. The general descriptions of the chapter sections follows:

Chapter Titles: The chapters are arranged alphabetically by subject matter. Subjects include *ailments*, such as HAYFEVER/ALLERGY, ARTHRITIS, and NAUSEA; *systems of the body*, such as the HEART, NERVES & GLANDS, and WHOLE BODY; *purposes*, such as CHOLESTEROL REGULATION, LAXATIVE, and WEIGHT LOSS; and *miscellaneous*, such as ENVIRONMENTAL POLLUTION.

Herbs: The herbs listed in this section can be used singly or, preferrably, in combination. The major herbs, or those with the more potent activity, are listed in Bold Upper Case. Other herbs may be potent on other occasions, or for other ailments, but for the particular condition(s) discussed in this chapter, they are meant to augment, modulate or otherwise modify the over all activity of the major herbs. In a blend these interactions would be more strongly felt.

Purpose and *Other Applications:* These sections list the conditions or purposes for which the herbs are intended in this chapter. Some conditons may seem unrelated to the chapter title, and are listed here to present an idea of the range of effects the herbs can possess.

Use: Compared to the orginal book, there are fewer uses listed in this section, mainly because much of the underlying supportive and coordinating information contained in the discussion has been edited out.

Contraindications: When herbs are selected properly, the potential for dangerous side effects, drug interactions and other hazards is very small. However, this section will list any cautions that should be taken with certain herbs. For example, diuretics have the potential of depleting the body's store of potassium and sometimes require that potassium supplements be taken.

Text: The body of the chapter contains information on the individual herbs. What information to include and what to edit out in these paragraphs was often a most difficult task. Generally, I have tried to retain a representative sampling of the kind of research that has transpired, a little flavor of the herb's heritage, and important notes on the herb's usage. Most often deleted kinds of information included discussions of the physiological causes and manifestations of disease or internal chemical processes, theoretical discussions of mode of action, repetative research data, and much clinical data. Make use of the chapter titles that appear at the end of each paragraph to find more information concerning that herb. Also use the index for this same purpose. The book is organized so that for every chapter's subject, only information on that subject is included in that chapter. Therefore, if the same herb occurs in more than one chapter, information about that herb in each chapter will be different.

References: The numbers in bold in the text are to the references that are listed in this section. These references are usually just a sample of those that can be found in **The Scientific Validation of Herbal Medicine**. Scientific data on the herbs in this book was drawn from standard medical journals published around the world. This information has remained largely unkown to the American public. Hopefully, this small book will change that.

NOTE: Many persons, on their first encounter with the information presented in this book, are tempted to throw out their medications and start using nothing but herbs. Please do not do that. Your education in this field is just beginning. In my opinion people should ease into the use of herbs, and ease out of the use of traditional medications, especially if their health problems are severe. A sudden switch of health regimen can be hazardous.

ARTHRITIS

HERBS: **ALFALFA seed & leaf** (*Medicago sativa*), **CELERY SEED** (*Apium graveolens*), **Burdock root** (*Arctium lappa*), **Chaparral** (*Larrea divaricata*), **Sarsaparilla Root** (*Smilax officinalis*), **Licorice root** (*Glycyrrhiza glabra*), **Kelp** (*Laminara, Macrocystis, Asocphyllum*), **Cayenne** (*Capsicum annum*), **Queen-of-the-Meadow root** (*Eupatorium purpureum*).

Form: Capsule, Tea, Poultice

PURPOSE: To help reduce symptoms such as stiff, inflamed and sore muscles and joints, due to Arthritis, Rheumatism, Lupus, Gout, and Bursitis.

Other Applications: Atherosclerosis, Blood Cleansing, Acidosis.

USE: 1. For General Use: 2 cap, 4 times per day, with 1/2 glass of liquid.
2. Prevention : 2-4 caps/day.
3. If used in conjunction with the WHOLE BODY TONIC Blend, reduce daily intact by 2 capsules and, for optimum results, increase the ENVIRONMENTAL POLLUTION Blend by two capsules.

Contraindications: None. Chaparral, although sometimes called creosote bush, contains **NO** creosote.

This blend's approach to arthritic ailments is to help reduce pain and inflammation while cleaning up and strengthening the blood, and while attempting to dissolve troublesome deposits in the joints.

ALFALFA's anti-rheumatic effect is probably due to its extremely high nutritive value. Alfalfa has a proven cholesterol lowering effect (**1**) and it generally helps to improve overall health, vigor and vitality (**2**); see also WHOLE BODY). Steroid properties are suggested by its saponin content, and by some research that shows an estrogenic effect in ruminants (grazing animals). Alfalfa, as fiber, is also good for cellular detoxification. *(See also ENVIRONMENTAL POLLUTION)*

CELERY SEED is a traditional diuretic and blood cleanser, well suited for treating rheumatism, especially when combined with Damiana (**3**). Its inclusion in arthritic blends is a rather modern tradition, but has repeatedly proven itself in clinical trials. A famous Chinese study showed that it lowered blood pressure in 14 of 16 human patients with chronic high blood pressure (**4**). In Europe, Celery Seed is a common medicinal treatment for gout and rheumatism (**5**). *(See also LIVER DISORDERS)*

BURDOCK ROOT is an effective blood purifier and pain killer. This property would partially explain its observed effectiveness in treating rheumatism. American herbalists have testified for the past two hundred years that Burdock can effectively alleviate symptoms of arthritis and other inflammatory diseases (**6**). *(See also BLOOD PURIFICATION/DETOXIFICATION; DETOXIFY/NURTURE; BONE-FLESH-CARTILAGE)*

CHAPARRAL, according to modern science and the best American Indian folklore, as well as modern science, has good anti-rheumatoid properties. The primary constituent of Chaparral, NDGA (nordihydroquaiaretic acid), possesses analgesic (pain relieving) and vasodepressant (circulatory depressing) properties (**7**); NDGA also increases ascorbic acid levels in the adrenals (**8**) and has antioxidant and anticancer activity (**9**). Finally, NDGA stimulates the process by which cells utilize foods for energy (**10**), a fact that may eventually provide the key to its effectiveness in treating arthritic conditions. *(See also SKIN; BONE-FLESH-CARTILAGE; DETOXIFY/NURTURE)*

SARSAPARILLA was independently discovered in the United States, as well as other countries around the world, to be an effective treatment for rheumatism (**11**). Mode of action may stem from its high content of saponins. *(See also INFERTILITY; DETOXIFY/NURTURE; WHOLE BODY; BLOOD PURIFICATION/DETOXIFICATION)*

LICORICE ROOT and its derivatives have been found to possess substantial anti-arthritic activity (**12**). This property is no doubt due to the herb's anti-inflammatory effects, although certain enzyme systems have also been implicated (**13**). The anti-inflammatory property of Licorice Root has been used in treating dermatological problems (**14**). In one study, the herb's derivatives were subjected to four established tests for anti-inflammatory properties. The tests results were positive on all counts (**15**). Since that time, several studies have been done to verify and extend those initial findings (e.g., **16**). The anti-inflammatory effect is probably related to a release of corticoids from the adrenals (**17**), because the effect seems to depend on an intact adrenal gland (**18**). The advantage in using Licorice Root is that it has none of the side effects associated with the use of glucocorticoid-type drugs such as cortisone and hydrocortisone. Yet Licorice Root and/or its derivatives can be every bit as effective as hydrocortisone (**16**). *(See also RESPIRATORY AILMENTS; SKIN; FEMALE TONIC; BLOOD PURIFICATION/DETOXIFICATION; CIRCULATION; FATIGUE; WEIGHT LOSS; ENVIRONMENTAL POLLUTION; FEVERS & INFECTIONS; THYROID; WHOLE BODY; DETOXIFY/NURTURE; MENTAL ALERTNESS/SENILITY)*

QUEEN-OF-THE-MEADOW herb has been established clinically as an effective treatment for rheumatic and gouty conditions caused by uric acid deposits in the joints (**19**). Because of its stimulating effect on glands and organs that clear the body of toxins and waste (**6**), it is also helpful in most forms of inflammatory distress. *(See also DIURETIC)*

KELP and **CAYENNE** provide nutritive support as well as improve good circulatory stimulation. They measurably enhance the overall effectiveness and usefulness of the blend. The trace mineral content of Kelp is among the highest of any source known, a fortunate circumstance for arthritic patients who use it.

OTHER NUTRIENTS

VITAMINS
(Daily requirements unless otherwise noted)
Vitamin A *25,000 I.U.*
Vitamin B Complex
Vitamin B1 *25-100 mg*
Vitamin B2 *25-100 mg*
Vitamin B6 *25-100 mg*
Vitamin B12 *4 mcg*
Vitamin C *3,000-4,000 mg*
Vitamin D *2,500 I.U.*
Vitamin E *600-800 I.U.*
Folic Acid Niacinamide *10 mg*
Pantothenic Acid *300 mg*

MINERALS
Calcium/Magnesium
Iodine
Phosphorous
Potassium
Sulfur
Manganese

MISCELLANEOUS
Lecithin
GLA
Essential Fatty Acid
Cod Liver Oil
HCl
Liver

REFERENCES

1. Malinow, M.R., McLaughlin, P., Papworth, M.S., Stafford, C., Kohler, G.O., Livingston, A.L., and Cheeke, P.R. "Effect of alfalfa saponins on intestinal cholesterol absorption in rats." **The American Journal of Clinical Nutrition.** 30 (Dec 1977), 2061-2067.
2. Ellingwood, F. **American Materia Medica, Therapeutics and Pharmacognosy.** Eclectic Medical Publications, Portland, Oregon, 1983.
3. List, P.H. & Hoerhammer, L. **Hagers Handbuch der Pharmazeutischen Praxis.** Volumes 2-5, Springer-Verlag, Berlin.
4. Grieve, M. **A Modern Herbal.** 2 vols. Hafner, New York, 1967.
5. Kiangsu Institute of Modern Medicine. **Encyclopedia of Chinese Drugs.** 2 Vols. Shanghai, Peoples Republic of China, 1977.
6. Felter, H. W. **The Eclectic Materia Medica, Pharmacology and Therapeutics.** Eclectic Medical Publications, Portland, Oregon, 1983 (first published 1922).
7. Bergel, M. "Nordihydroquaiaretic acid in therapy." **Semana Medical.** (Buenos Aires), II, 123-131, 1955.
8. Sporn, A. & Schobesch, O. "Toxicity of nordihyroguaiaretic acid." **Igiena** (Bucharest), 15(12), 725-726, 1966.
9. Waller, C. W. & Gisvold, O. N. "A phytochemical investigation of Larrea Divaricata Cav." **Journal Of the American Pharmaceutical Association,** 34, 78-81, 1945.
10. Scharff, M. & Wilson, R.H. "Nordihydroguaiaretic acid effects on the metabolism of mung beam mitochondria." **Plant & cell Physiology.** 16, 865-869, 1975.
11. Leung, A.Y. **Encyclopedia of Common Natural Ingredients.** New York, 1980.
12. Tangri, K.K., Seth, P.K. Parmar, S.S. & Bhargava, K.P. "Biochemical study of anti-inflammatory and anti-arthritic properties of glycyrrhetic acid." **Biochemical Pharmacology,** 14(8), 1277-1281, 1965.
13. Parmar, S.S., Tangri, K.K., Seth, P.K. & Bhargava, K.P. "Biochemical basis for anti-inflammatory effects of glycyrrhetic acid and its derivatives." **International Congress of Biochemistry,** 6(5), 410, 1967.
14. Adamson, A.C. & Tillman, W.G. "Hydrocortisone." **British Medical Journal.,** 2, 1501, 1955.
15. Kumagi, A., Yano, S., & Otomo, M. "The corticoid-like action of glycyrrhizin and the mechanism of its action." **Endocrinologia Japonica,** 4, 17-21, 1961.
16. Finney, S.H., & Somers, G.F. "The anti-inflammatory activity of glycyrrhetinic acid and derivatives." **Journal of Pharmacology and Pharmacodynamics.** 10(10), 613-620, 1958.
17. Tamura, Y. "Study of effects of glycyrrhetinic acid and its derivatives on delta 4-5 alpha and 5 beta-reductase by rat liver preparations." **Folia Endocrinologia Japonica,** 51(7), 589-600, 1975.
18. Gibson, M.R. "Glycyrrhiza in old and new perspective." **Lloydia,** 41(4), 348-354, 1978.
19. Hutchens, A.R. **Indian Herbalogy of North America.** Merco, Ontario, Canada, 1969.

HIGH BLOOD PRESSURE

HERBS: GARLIC (*Allium sativum*), **VALERIAN** root (*Valeriana officinalis*), **Black Cohosh root** (*Cimicifuga racemosa*), **Cayenne** (*Capsicum annum*), & **Kelp** (*Laminara, Macrocystis, Ascophyllum*).

Form: Capsule.

PURPOSE: High blood pressure (Hypertension); any condition that may be aggravated by nervous anxiety; To reduce serum cholesterol.

Other Applications: Hives, Shingles, Erysipelas, Insomnia.

USE: 1. Anxiety attacks: 4 caps, 3 times per day
2. Prevention: 3-5 capsper day
3. High blood pressure: 2-3 caps, 3-4 times per day
4. To assist the body in maintaining proper blood cholesterol levels: 4 capsules daily, in conjunction with the CHOLESTEROL REGULATION Blend.
5. To supplement the NERVOUS TENSION Blend: 2-4 caps/day.

Contraindications: None.

Hypertension is a hybrid of physiological, emotional and mental factors. Physiologically, it is often aggravated by athero- and arteriosclerosis, obesity and drug abuse (including cigarettes, alcohol and caffeine). Emotionally and mentally, hypertension normally occurs in persons with stressful lifestyles, characterized by worry, hurry and flurry. This blend seeks to reduce blood cholesterol levels, hypertension and anxiety. People suffering from hypertension, nervous anxiety and the stress of modern living will find this blend a valuable adjunct to their lifestyles—and their health.

GARLIC possesses nearly two dozen major medicinal properties. Two of those are important in this blend: the ability to lower blood cholesterol levels and a hypotensive property. Garlic contains several volatile sulphur compounds (like allicin) which are the probable active constituents. Animal and human basic research has irrefutably established Garlic's ability to lower blood serum cholesterol levels (**1-2**). The typical study compares diets high in fat with and without Garlic. Garlic diets consistently produce the lowest cholesterol levels (**3**). In one study, 40 of 100 patients with high blood pressure experienced a reduction of 20 mmHg or more after about a week of Garlic treatment (**4**). In animal studies the herb significantly lowers blood cholesterol levels (up to 80%) (e.g., **5**). Extrapolating from the data, it can be concluded that regular Garlic ingestion could have dramatic beneficial effects of the course of heart disease due to atherosclerosis. When humans are matched as to age and sex, there are significant differences between those that eat Garlic and onion and those that don't, manifested in factors which influence the course of atherosclerosis. For example, those who use Garlic and onion have much lower serum-triglycerides, beta lipoproteins, phospholipids and plasma fibrinogen levels (**6**). Another important property of Garlic is its hypotensive activity. Rabbits and humans who have been given Garlic show a rapid and prolonged decrease in blood pressure (**7**). Finally, Garlic inhibits the tendency of blood cells to stick together (platelet aggregation), thereby reducing the tendency toward hypertension (**8**). *(See also FEVERS & INFECTIONS; PARASITES)*

BLACK COHOSH has been one the favorite herbs of Americans for at least two centuries. Some pharmacological investigation conducted on this plant has confirmed its hypotensive and vasodilatory effects (**9-10**). These findings, from America, China and Europe, validate Black Cohosh's reputation as a sedative and hypotensive. In Europe, it is believed that the herb exhibits hypotensive properties by inhibiting the vasomotor centers in the central nervous system (**11**). *(See also FEMALE TONIC; NERVOUS TENSION)*

CAYENNE will also lower blood cholesterol levels, thereby helping to reduce blood pressure . In one study (**12**), separate groups of rats were fed diets high in cholesterol with or without ground Cayenne or capsaicin, the active constituent of Cayenne, for seven weeks. Both Cayenne and capsaicin prevented rise in liver cholesterol levels, and increased fecal excretions of free cholesterol. These findings show that Cayenne prevents even the absorption of cholesterol. Cayenne also reduces the blood pressure in an even more direct manner: a number of years ago, a team of researchers discovered that capsaicin acts in a reflexive manner to reduce systemic blood pressure, a kind of coronary chemoreflex (**13**). *(See also CIRCULATION; BLOOD PURIFICATION/DETOXIFICATION; FATIGUE)*

VALERIAN ROOT is one of the most studied plants. Valerian and/or its major constituents, the valepotriates, have marked sedative, anticonvulsive, hypotensive, tranquilizing, neurotropic, and anti-aggressive properties (e.g., **14-15**). These effects result from a selective neurotropic action of the root on higher brain centers. The herb's main functional effect is to suppress and regulate the autonomic nervous system. As a result, it has been found effective in treating psychosomatic diseases and childhood behavioral disorders that involve dysregulation of the autonomic nervous system. Many forms of restlessness and tension also yield to the effects of Valerian root. *(See also NERVOUS TENSION; INSOMNIA)*

KELP's considerable hypotensive activity is discussed in the HEART chapter.

OTHER NUTRIENTS

VITAMINS
(Daily requirements unless otherwise noted)
Vitamin B Complex-High Potency
Vitamin B6 *25 mg*
Vitamin C *1,000-3,000 mg*
Vitamin E *200-600 I.U.*
Choline 1,000 mg
Inositol 1,000 mg
Niacinamide *100 mg*
Bioflavanoids *100-300 mg*

MINERALS
Calcium/Magnesium
Potassium
Phosphorous

MISCELLANEOUS
GLA
Essential Fatty Acid
Cod Liver Oil
Brewer's Yeast
Lecithin
Wheat Germ
Liver

REFERENCES

1. Sial, A.Y. & Ahmed, S.I. "Study of the hypotensive action of garlic extract in experimental animals." **Journal of the Pakistan Medical Association.** 32(10), 237-239, 1982.

2. Kamanna, V.S. & Chandrasekhara, N. "Effect of garlic on serum lipoproteins and lipoprotein cholesterol levels in albino rats rendered hypercholesteremic by feeding cholesterol." **Lipids.** 17(7), 483-488, 1982.

3. Bordia. A. & Bansal, H.C. "Essential oil of garlic in prevention of atherosclerosis." **The Lancet.** II, 1491, 1973.

4. Piotrowski, G. "L'ail en therapeutique." **Praxis**, 37, 488-492, 1948.

5. Bordia, A., Arora, S.K., Kothori, L.K., et.al. "The protective action of essential oils of onion and garlic in cholesterol-fed rabbits." **Atherosclerosis**, 22, 103-109, 1975.

6. Sainani, G.S., Desai, D.B. & More, K.N. "Onion, garlic and atherosclerosis." **The Lancet**, Sept 11, 575-576, 1976.7. Korotkov, V.M. "The action of garlic juice on blood pressure." **Vrachebnoe Delo**, 6, 123, 1966.

8. Srivastava, K.C. "Effects of aqueous extracts of onion, garlic and ginger on platelet aggregation and metabolism of arachidonic acid in blood vascular system: In vitro study." **Prostaglandins Leukotrienes and Medicine**, 13, 227-235, 1984.

9. Macht, D.I. & Cook, H.M. "A pharmacological note on cimicifuga." **Journal of the American Pharmaceutical Association.** 21(4), 324-330, 1932. (It was on the basis of many negative findings in this study, that research on the herb was abandoned and it fell into disrepute in traditional medicine in the U.S.A.)

10. Genazzani, E. & Sorrentino, L. "Vascular action of acteina: active constituent of actaea racemosa L." **Nature.** 194(4828), 544-545, 1962.

11. List, P.H. & Hoerhammer, L. **Hagers Handbuch der Pharmazeutischen Praxis.** Volumes 2-5, Springer-Verlag, Berlin.

12. Sambaiah, K. & Satyanarayana, M.N. "Hypocholesterolemic effect of red pepper & capsaicin." **Indian Journal of Experimental Biology.** 18 (8), 898-899, 1980.

13. Toh, C.C., Lee, T.S. & Kiang, A.K. "The pharmacological actions of capsaicin and analogues." **British Journal of Pharmacology.** 10, 175-182, 1955.

14. Gstirner, F. & Kleinbauer, E. "Zur pharmakologischen Pruefung der Baldrianwurzel." (Toward the pharmacological examination of Valerian root). **Pharmazie.** 13(7), 416-419, 1958.

15. Hauschild, F. "Die problematik der sedativen baldrianwirkung." **Pharmazie.** 13(7), 420-422, 1958.

BLOOD PURIFICATION AND DETOXIFICATION

HERBS: DANDELION root (*Taraxacum officinale*), YELLOW DOCK root (*Rumex crispus*), **Sarsaparilla root** (*Smilax officinalis*), **Echinacea** (*Echinacea purpurea*), **Licorice root** (*Glycyrrhiza glabra*), **Cayenne** (*Capsicum annum*), & **Kelp** (*Laminaria, Macrocystis, Ascophyllum*).

Form: Capsule, Tea

PURPOSE: Blood purifier and detoxifier. By itself or to support several other blends.

Other Applications: Acne, obesity, gout, moles, viral warts, body odor, venereal disease, general toxicity, skin sores and swellings, skin cancer, endocrine and exocrine gland disorders.

USE: 1. Detoxification, purification & cleansing programs: 3-4 caps, 2-3 times per day, with meals.
2. To support the problems discussed under ARTHRITIS, SKIN DISORDERS, and FEVERS & INFECTIONS. and 29: 1 cap, 3 times per day with meals.
3. Routine Maintenance: 2-4 caps daily with meals.
4. To help treat liver problems (see LIVER DISORDERS): 2 caps, four times per day, never on empty stomach.

Contraindications: None.

It is difficult to overestimate the importance of maintaining a healthy supply of blood. The blood performs many vital functions which sometimes become overtaxed during acute and chronic cellular disease. Likewise, many ailments and diseases are the result of impurities and toxins in the blood. The blood is therefore a target for effective medicinal intervention. This blend could properly be termed an "alterative," meaning that it gradually changes the properties of the blood from unhealthy to healthy. What happens is toxins and wastes are filtered out, microbial poisons are killed, vital salts are adjusted and balanced, nutrients are furnished, and important plasma substances are strengthened and enhanced. You may use this blend for the ailments listed under *Other Applications*, or whenever your symptoms include ugly sores, easy bruising, mucous diseased gums, exhaustion, anemia, cancer, venereal disease, and related conditions.

DANDELION ROOT acts by straining and filtering toxins and wastes from the bloodstream. A complete discussion of Dandelion's effects on liver function is presented in the chapters on DIABETES and LIVER DISORDERS. It is important to note here that the herb has been shown to uniformly remedy chronic liver congestion (**1**). and has been used in medical practice to successfully treat hepatitis, swelling of the liver, jaundice and dyspepsia with deficient bile secretion (**2**). (See also NERVES & GLANDS; SKIN DISORDERS; DIABETES; LIVER DISORDERS)

YELLOW DOCK increases the ability of the liver and related organs to strain and purify the blood. Formerly, Yellow Dock was a primary treatment for scurvy and anemia. The eclectics used it often when they felt that some particular skin disease was caused by blood-borne toxins (see the chapter on SKIN DISORDERS). To this day the herb is an important ingredient in alterative preparations in European countries (e.g., Germany, Russia, France, England and Switzerland), North American countries, China and India. (See also SKIN DISORDERS)

SARSAPARILLA root actually attacks microbial substances in the blood stream, neutralizing them (**3**). This effect is primarily due to the plant's antibiotic principles. (**4**). The herb is also a strong diuretic, thereby stimulating the excretion of wastes such as uric acid and excess chloride. To a lesser degree the plant is a diaphoretic—by promoting sweating still more toxins are removed from the lymph and circulatory systems. Psoriasis is especially vulnerable to the effects of Sarsaparilla. (See also INFERTILITY; ARTHRITIS; WHOLE BODY; DETOXIFY/NURTURE)

LICORICE root acts in an extremely complex manner to adjust the concentrations of vital blood salts, thereby stimulating and sustaining proper adrenal function (**5**). Licorice root protects the blood supply and enhances its purity by protecting the body's blood detoxification plant—the liver, from serious diseases, such as cirrhosis (**6**) and hepatitis (**7**).

CAYENNE is primarily a kind of catalyst in the blood purification process. It stimulates the vital organs to greater activity, promotes cardiovascular activity, while lowering overall blood pressure (**8**). But additionally, it acts directly as a diaphoretic, stimulating excretion of wastes in the sweat. (See also CIRCULATION; HIGH BLOOD PRESSURE; FATIGUE; INFLUENZA)

KELP is a general nutritive tonic to the blood, supplying essential vitamins and mineral salts. Kelp is an important adjunct to any cleansing program since it can bind radioactive strontium, barium, cadmium and zinc, some of our most dangerous pollutants, in the gastrointestinal tract, thus preventing their absorption into the body (**9**). It has been postulated that Kelp may activate the body's immune system (**10**) (see chapter DEGENERATIVE DISORDERS for details). If proven true, this may explain some of Kelp's remarkable alterative properties. Kelp is neither carcinogenic nor toxic.

BURDOCK root comes about as close to a good old fashioned alterative or blood cleanser as anything in this blend. Thus, it produces gradual beneficial changes in the body by improving general nutrition and by gradually altering the health of the blood. It is both diuretic and diaphoretic. Burdock has been shown to enhance liver and bile functions (**11**). Bacteriostatic principles have been isolated from Burdock (**12**), and it has been found to inhibit tumor growth (**13**). (See also DETOXIFY/NURTURE; SKIN DISORDERS; BONE-FLESH-CARTILAGE)

ECHINACEA is also a classical alterative. The therapeutic use of Echinacea can be traced to the North American Indians who used it to heal wounds, for insect and snake bites, to combat infections, both externally and internally. Clinically, this herb can be expected to stimulate most of the glands and glandular organs (esp. the kidneys) to greater and more efficient activity. Digestion, absorption, assimilation, resorption, secretion and excretion are all promoted in a concerted effort to prevent auto-intoxication. In an important study bearing on these properties, Echinacea has been found to increase the phagocytic activity of leukocytes (the ability of white blood cells to fight, destroy and eat toxic organisms that invade the body) (**14**). (See also SKIN DISORDERS; FEVERS & INFECTIONS)

OTHER NUTRIENTS

VITAMINS
(Daily requirements unless otherwise noted)

Vitamin A *25,000 I.U. (25,000 I.U. for short intervals)*	
Vitamin B Complex	
Vitamin B2 *25-100 mg*	Niacinamide *100 mg*
Vitamin B-6 *25-50 mg*	Pantothenic Acid *50-100 mg*
Vitamin B-12 *25 mg*	Choline *500-1000 mg*
Vitamin C *500-1,000 mg*	Inositol *500-600 mg*
Vitamin D *200-400 I.U.*	PABA *10 mg*
Vitamin E *200-600 I.Y.*	Folic acid *400 mcg*

MINERALS
Potassium Calcium/Magnesium

REFERENCES

1. Leclerc, H. **Phytotherapie (Paris)**, 1927, cited by Ripperger, W. "Pflanzliche laxantien und cholagogue wirkungen." **Medizinische Welt**, 9, 1463, 1935.
2. Kroeber, L. "Pharmacology of inulin drugs and their therapeutic use. II. Cichorium intybus; taraxacum officinale. **Pharmazie**, 5, 122-127, 1950.
3. Tschesche, R. "Advances in the chemistry of antibiotic substances from higher plants." in Wagner, H. & Horhammer, L. **Pharmacognosy and Phytochemistry**. Springer Verlag, N.Y. 1971, pp. 274-276.
4. D'Amico. "Richerche sulla presenza di sostanze ad azione antibiotica nelle piante superiori." **Fitoterapia**. 21(1), 1950, 77-79.
5. Kumagi, A, Asanuman, U., Yano, S., Takevchik, Morimoto, Y., Vemura, T. & Yamamura, Y. "Effect of glycyrrhizin on the suppressive action of cortisone on the pituitary adrenal axis." **Endocrinologia Japonica**, 13, 235-244, 1966.
6. Zhao, M., Han, D., Ma, X., Zhao, Y., Yin, L. & Li, C. "The preventive and therapeutic actions of glycyrrhizin, glycyrrhetic acid and crude saikosides on experimental cirrhosis in rats." **Yao Hsueh Hsueh Pao**, 18(5), 325-331, 1983.
7. Fujisawa, K., Watanabe, Y. * Kimura, K. "Therapeutic approach to chronic active hepatitis with glycyrrhizin." **Asian Medical Journal**, 23, 745-756, 1980.
8. de Lille, J. & Ramirez, E. "Pharmacodynamic action of the active principles of chillie (capsicum annuum L)." **Anales Inst. Biol.**, 6, 23-37, 1935.
9. Tanaka, Y., Hurlburt, A.J., Argeloff, L., Skoryna, S.C. & Stara, J.F. "Application of algal polysaccharides as in vivo binders of metal pollutants." in **Proceedings of the Seventh International Seaweed Symposium**, Wiley & Sons, N.Y., 602-607, 1972.
10. Taylor, W.A., Sheldon, D., & Spicer, J.W. "Adjuvant and suppressive effects of grass conjuvac and other alginate conjugates on IgG and IgE antibody responses in mice." **Immunology**, 44, 41-50, 1981.
11. Chabrol, E. & Charonnat, R. "Therapeutic agents in bile secretion." **Ann. Med.**, 37, 131-142, 1935.
12. Foldeak, S. & Dombradi, G.A. "Tumor-growth inhibiting substances of plant origin. I. Isolation of the active principle of arctium lappa." **Acta Univ. Szeged., Phys. Chem.**, 10, 91-93, 1964.
13. Schulte, K.E., Ruecker, G. & Perlick, J. "polyacetylene compounds in Echinacea purpurea and e. augustifolia." **Arzneimittel Forschungen**, 17(7), 825-829, 1967.
14. Ellingwood, F. **American Materia Medica, Therapeutics and Pharmacognosy**. Eclectic Medical Publications, Portland, Oregon, 1983.

LOW BLOOD SUGAR

HERBS: **LICORICE** root (*Glycyrrhiza glabra*), **GOTU KOLA** (*Hydrocotyle asiatica*), **Siberian Ginseng** (*Eleutherococcus senticosus*), & **Ginger** (*Zingiber officinale*).

Form: Tea, Capsule.

PURPOSE: To counter the effects of low blood sugar and to support glucose metabolism.

Other Applications: Fatigue, Exhaustion, Adrenal Exhaustion.

USE: 1. Anywhere from 4 to 8 capsules per day can be recommended depending on the severity of symptoms.
2. To supplement the FATIGUE Blend: 4 capsules per day.
3. To supplement the MENTAL ALERTNESS/SENILITY Blend: 3-4 capsules per day.

Contraindications: Some forms of low blood sugar involve very low serum potassium levels. Please have your physician check your potassium. If it is low, be sure to supplement the use of this blend with potassium tablets.

Low blood sugar may result from any one of several conditions: 1) Overproduction of insulin; 2) Damage to liver cells; 3) Insufficient secretion of adrenocortical hormones; and 4) Pituitary gland abnormalities. This blend is designed to remedy cause 3 above. Since the effects of stress are felt mainly by the adrenals, it is probable that most cases of hypoglycemia are of this type. Prolonged hypoglycemia that resists the measures presented here should be treated by a competent physician. "Functional" hypoglycemia, due to severe muscular exertion, poor nutrition and other stressors, will yield nicely to the tonic effects of this blend.

*LICORICE ROOT*s role in treating hypoglycemia is to increase the effectiveness of glucocorticoids (adrenal hormones) circulating in the liver, and to mimic the action of these hormones itself (**1-2**). This mechanism would work in cases of low blood sugar brought on by adrenal stress. Often the adrenals simply cannot keep up with the demands of stress on the body. Licorice root can help to reverse the symptoms, but long term health maintenance demands better overall nutrition at the very least. Complete adrenal exhaustion is known as Addison's disease. In this condition none of the three major classes of adrenalcortical hormones are being produced. Some rather severe problems develop. Licorice root constituents have been shown to help the body overcome adrenal failure, which could lead to Addison's disease (**3-4**). Their effectiveness derives from their ability to maintain the proper electrolyte balance in tissues (normally the role of aldosterone), and from their ability to prevent the enzymatic destruction of whatever glucocorticoids and mineralcorticoids happen to be present in the cells (**3-8**), thus allowing these hormones to circulate and be active longer. *(See also DETOXIFY/NURTURE; FEMALE TONIC; WHOLE BODY; FEVERS & INFECTIONS; INFERTILITY;ARTHRITIS; SKIN DISORDERS; BLOOD PURIFICATION/DETOXIFICATION; CIRCULATION; WEIGHT LOSS; ENVIRONMENTAL POLLUTION; MENTAL ALERTNESS/SENILITY)*

GOTU KOLA is used to build up good adrenal health. See the chapters on FATIGUE, WHOLE BODY TONIC, and MENTAL ALERTNESS/SENILITY for discussions of this herb.

SIBERIAN GINSENG, through the interplay of its many active constituents, including the panaxosides and ginsengosides, is often able to *normalize* physiological imbalances (**9**). In this case, research has shown that it can raise abnormally low blood sugar levels (**10**) and that it can lower abnormally high blood sugar levels (**11**). Ginseng's effect on blood sugar levels is probably the indirect result of its effect on the total organism. Since a person suffering from hyperglycemia or hypoglycemia presents a complex picture of physiological symptoms, including deficiencies and excesses, any agent that improves general cellular health will have a positive effect on both conditions. And this is exactly what Ginseng does (e.g., **12-13**). *(See also INFERTILITY; FATIGUE; WHOLE BODY TONIC; MENTAL ALERTNESS/SENILITY)*

GINGER ROOT probably does not have a direct effect on blood sugar levels. Nevertheless, it is an important herb for hypoglycemics to use. It works indirectly to increase the availability of dietary nutrients for digestion and metabolism. Whenever the hypoglycemic condition is attended and/or made worse by improper digestion and assimilation of foods, Ginger root will markedly facilitate the utilization of energy stores (**14**). Functional hypoglycemia, that rundown feeling, is especially well-served by this treatment. *(See also CIRCULATION; NERVOUS TENSION; FATIGUE; DIGESTION; NAUSEA; STOMACH/INTESTINAL)*

OTHER NUTRIENTS

VITAMINS
(Daily requirements unless otherwise noted)
Vitamin B Complex
Vitamin B1 *25-50 mg*
Vitamin B2 *25-50 mg*
Vitamin B6 *25-50 mg*
Vitamin B12 *25-50 mg*
Pantothenic acid *100-200 mg*
Vitamin C *2,000-5,000 mg*
Vitamin E *600-800 I.U.*

MINERALS
Calcium/Magnesium
Phosphorous
Chromium
Potassium

MISCELLANEOUS
HCl
Brewer's yeast

REFERENCES

1. Tamura, Y. "Study of effects of glycyrrhetinic acid and its derivatives on 4-5 alpha and beta-reductase by rat liver preparations." **Folia Endocrinologia Japonica**, 8, 164-188, 1975.
2. Kumagai, A, Asanuman, U., Yano, S., Takevchik, Morimoto, Y., Vemura, T., & Yamamura, Y. "Effect of glycyrrhizin on the suppressive action of cortisone on the pituitary adrenal axis." **Endocrinologia Japonica**, 13, 235-244, 1966.
3. Borst, J.G.G., Ten Holt, S.P., de Vries, L.A., & Molhuysen, J.A. "Synergistic action of liquirice and cortisone in Addison's and Simmond's disease." **Lancet**, 1, 657-663, 1953.
4. Pelser, H.E., Willerbrands, A.F., Frenkel, M., van der Heide, & Groen, J. "Comparative study of the use of glycyrrhizinic and glycyrrhetinic acids in Addison's Disease." **Metabolism**, 2, 322-334, 1953.
5. Card, J., Strong, J.A., Tompsett, M.W., Taylor, N.R.W. & Wilson, J.M.G. "Effects of liquorice and its derivatives on salt and water metabolism." **Lancet**, 1, 663-668, 1953.
6. Groen, J. Pelser, H.E., Frenkel, M., Wilderbrands, A.F. & Kamminga, C.E. "Extracts of glycyrrhizinic acid on the electrolyte metabolism in Addison's disease." **Journal of Clinical Investigations**, 31, 87-91, 1952.
7. Armanini, D., Karbowiak, I. & Fulder, J.W. "Affinity of liquorice derivatives for mineralcorticoid and glucocorticoid receptors." **Clinical Endocrinology** (Oxf), 19(5), 609-612, 1983.
8. Tamura, Y., Nishikawa, K., Yamada, M, Yamamotoa, M. & Kumagi, A. "Effects of glycyrrhetinic acid and its derivatives on delta-four-5-alpha and 5-beta reductase in rat liver." **Arzneimittel-Forschung.**, 29(4), 647-649, 1979.
9. Cheng-chia, L. & Ching-ch'u, T. "Successful treatment of postpartum hypopituitarism with decoction of radix glycyrrhizae and radix ginseng." **Chinese Medical Journal**, 11, 156, 1973.
10. Fulder, S. "Ginseng: useless root or subtle medicine." **New Scientist**, 73(1035), 138-139, 1977.
11. Waki, I., Kyo, H., Yasuda, M., Kimura, M. "Effects of a hypoglycemic component of ginseng radix on insulin biosynthesis in normal and diabetic animals." **Journal of Pharmacobio-dynamics**, 5(8), 547-549, 1982.
12. Jiang, J., Zhang, Z., Zhang, L. & Huang, M. "Effects of general saponin of panax notoginseng and sanchinoside C-1 on blood sugar in experimental animals." **Acta Pharmaceutica Sinica (Yao Hsueh Hsueh Pao)**, 17(3), 222-225, 1982.
13. Yokozawa, T., Seno, H., Oura, H. "Effect of ginseng extract on lipid and sugar metabolism. I. Metabolic correlation between liver and adipose tissue." **Chemical and Pharmaceutical Bulletin**, Tokyo, 23, 3095-3100, 1975.
14. Iijima, M. & Higashi, T. "Effect of ginseng saponins on nuclear ribionucleic acid (rna) metabolism. II. RNA polymerase activities in rats treated with ginsenoside." **Chem. Pharm. Bull.**, 27(9), 2130-2136, 1979.
15. Oura, H., Tsukadea, K. & Nakagawa, H. "Effect of radix ginseng on cytoplasmic polysomes in the rat liver." **Chemical and Pharmaceutical Bulletin**, 20(2), 219-225, 1972.
16. Sakakibara, K., Shibata, Y., Tokuhiko, H., Sanada, S. & Shoji, J. "Effect of ginseng saponins on cholesterol metabolism. I. Level and the synthesis of serum and liver cholesterol in rats treated with ginsenosides." **Chemical and Pharmaceutical Bulletin**, 23(5), 1009-1016, 1975.
17. Oura, H., Hiai, S., Odaka, Y. & Yokozawa, T. "Studies on the biochemical action of ginseng saponin. I. purification from ginseng extract of the active component stimulating serum protein biosynthesis." **Journal of Biochemistry**, 77(5), 1057-1065, 1975.
18. Thompson, E.H., Wolk, I.D. & Allen, C.E. "Ginger rhizome: a new source of proteolytic enzyme." **Journal of Food Science**, 38(4), 652-655, 1973.
19. Glatzel, H. "Treatment of dyspetic disorders with spice extracts." **Hippokrates**, 40(23), 916-919, 1969.

BONE-FLESH-CARTILAGE SUPPLEMENT

HERBS: HORSETAIL (*Equisetum arvense*), **CHAPARRAL** (*Larrea divaricata*) **Parsley** (*Petroselinum sativum*), **Burdock** (*Arctium lappa*), **Marshmallow** (*Althea officinalis*), **Slippery Elm** (*Ulmus vulva*), **Plantain** (*Plantago ovata*).

Form: Capsule, Poultice, Compress, Mouthwash

PURPOSE: To provide nutritive support for bones, skin and related tissue, and to promote tissue healing.

Other Applications: Arthritis, Bursitis, Rheumatism.

USE: 1. Internal: 4-8 caps per day. Use more if severe injury or other conditions warrant.
2. External: 4 caps for small areas. 8 caps for larger areas. Apply as poultice or compress.

Contraindications: None. Chaparral contains **no** creosote.

Herbs can supply many important nutrients, as well as active principles, that heal, soothe and remedy skin, bones and connective tissue, both internally and externally. Several of the herbs in this blend contain large quantities of more or less inert mucilage that cleans and sanitizes wounds, absorbing toxins from sores and wounds, both inside and outside the body.

HORSETAIL or **SHAVEGRASS** has been shown to possess hemolytic (blood clotting) (**1**) and antibiotic (**2**) activity, properties that contribute to the healing process. Horsetail also supplies calcium and is rich in several other minerals that the body uses to rebuild injured tissue. Externally, Horsetail can be applied as a poultice.

CHAPARRAL has substantial clinical and experimental support as a treatment for skin cancer (see DETOXIFY/NURTURE for details). NDGA (nordihydroquaiaretic acid), the primary constituent of Chaparral, has been shown to significantly inhibit the formation of dental caries (**3**). There is also research that indicates that Chaparral helps reduce inflammation (**4**), and inhibits forms of pathogenic organisms. These data, together with those discussed in other chapters, clearly indicate that Chaparral plays an important role in healing skin and bone tissue, and in preventing pathogenic damage. *(See also SKIN DISORDERS; ARTHRITIS; DETOXIFY/NURTURE)*

PARSLEY serves two functions in this blend. First it imparts a measure of essential oil that invigorates the body, its blood supply and its tissues. Secondly, it supplies a good deal of nutrients. Its protein content (needed in the mending of bones) is over 20%, and it contains vitamins A, C, B-complex and K. Parsley is also hypotensive and bacteriostatic. *(See also DIURETIC; DIABETES; PROSTATE)*

BURDOCK, is in this blend because the skin and bones need a pure supply of blood in order to heal properly. The heart benefits from the presence of inulin in Burdock, since this substance is a source of the sugar fructose which is converted by the liver more rapidly into glycogen than other sugars. Burdock is high in the healing B vitamins and vitamin C. It possess activity against tumor growth (**9**), and is a natural antibiotic. *(See also BLOOD PURIFICATION/DETOXIFICATION; DETOXIFY/NURTURE; SKIN DISORDERS)*

MARSHMALLOW soothes mucous membranes, and has been used externally for hundreds of years as a wound healer. Mainly, it is used internally to treat inflammation and mucosal afflictions of the genito-urinary tract. It is also used to soothe an irritated respiratory tract. It is used as a mouthwash and gargle and for helping infants cut new teeth (**1, 6**).

SLIPPERY ELM never became a truly popular herb until the English settlers noticed its widespread use by the Indians. Since then, medical botanists have never given up using Slippery Elm bark for just about any condition involving injured or infected tissue and bone (**7**). *(See also HEMORRHOIDS/ASTRINGENT; RESPIRATORY AILMENTS)*

PLANTAIN provides mucilaginous substance that contains healing properties that other mucilaginous plants do not possess. For example, people with poison ivy dermatitis have been treated with Plantain leaf, after which the itching immediately subsided and did not return (**8**). Most early American Physicians used Plantain for any skin infection or inflammation, and the treatment still meets with success.

OTHER NUTRIENTS

VITAMINS
(Daily requirement unless otherwise noted)
Vitamin A *25,000 I.U.*
Vitamin B ComplexVitamin B1 *50 mg*
Vitamin B2 *50 mg*
Vitamin B6 *50 mg*
Vitamin B12 *30-900 mcg*
Vitamin C *500-1,000 mg*
Vitamin D *800-3,000 I.U.*
Vitamin E *600-800 I.U.*
Pantothenic acid *150 mg*

MINERALS
Calcium/Magnesium
Phosphorous
Copper

MISCELLANEOUS
HCl

REFERENCES

1. List, P.H. & Hoerhammer, L. **Hagers Handbuch der Pharmazeutischen Praxis.** Volumes 2-5, Springer-Verlag, Berlin.
2. Sommer, L., Mintzer, L. & Rindasu, G. "Antimicrobial activity of the volatile oil extracted from equisetum arvense." **Farmacia Bucharest.**, 10, 535-541, 1962.
3. Lisanti, V.F. & Eichel, B. "Antioxidant inhibition of experimental induced caries." **Journal of Dental Research**, 42, 1030-1035, 1963.
4. Sporn, A. & Schobesch, O. "Toxicity of nordihydroquaiaretic acid." **Igiena**, (Bucharest), 15(12), 725-726, 1966.
5. Foldeak, S. & Dombradi, G.A. "Tumor-growth inhibiting substances of plant origin. I. Isolation of the active principle of arctium lappa." **Acta Physiology and Chemistry (Szeged)**, 10, 91-93, 1964.
6. Schauenberg, P. & Paris, F. **Guide des plantes medicinales**, Delachaux et Niestle, S.A., Neuchatel, Switzerland, 1969.
7. Gunn, J.D. **New Domestic Physician or Home Book of Health**, Moore, Wilstach, Keys. Cincinnati, 1st ed., 1857, 2nd ed 1859, 3rd ed 1961.
8. Duckett, S. "Plantain leaf for poison ivy." **Lancet**, 303(10), 583, 1980.

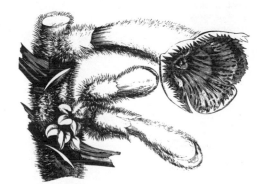

CHOLESTEROL REGULATION

HERBS: APPLE PECTIN, Hawthorn berries (*Crataegus oxyacantha*), **Plantain** (*Plantago ovata*), **Fenugreek** (*Trigonella Foenum-graecum*), **Black Cohosh root** (*Cimicifuga racemosa*), & **Cayenne** (*Capsicum annum*).

Form: Capsule.

PURPOSE: To help the body lower high serum cholesterol; to help prevent the deposition of dietary cholesterol on arterial walls.

Other Applications: To reduce the risk of debilitating disease. A dieting aid.

USE:
1. To reduce or reverse cholesterol build up: 1-2 caps per meal
2. For acute conditions: 4-6 caps/day.
3. Dieting aid: 1 cap per meal (with WEIGHT LOSS blend).
4. Use with HEART blend and HIGH BLOOD PRESSURE blend to increase their effectiveness.

Contraindications: None. Insulin-requiring diabetics should inform their physicians (see Pectin below). Hawthorn may potentiate the action of digitalis. Advise your physician if you are using both.

Cholesterol is a waxy, white substance that is classified as a fat, and is essential to life. However, it may accumulate on the arterial walls, dangerously constricting the flow of blood. Herbs can help reduce cholesterol levels, and reduce the risk of heart disease and atherosclerosis. This blend provides a high concentration of herbs with known cholesterol-lowering action in a base of other herbs which, in homeopathic doses, help tone the entire circulatory system, providing nutrition, strength and vitality.

PECTIN, in the diets of humans and lab animals, has been shown to increase the excretion of lipids, cholesterol and bile acids, and reduce serum cholesterol levels (**1-2**). Pectins may operate by binding with bile acids, thereby decreasing cholesterol and fat absorption (**3**). Pectin is also effective in causing regressions in, and preventing, gallstones (**4**). There is also evidence that the regular use of Pectin may lessen the severity of diabetes (**5**). Along these lines, it has been suggested that fiber-depleted diets actually help cause diabetes mellitus (**6**). Other studies have shown that fiber and pectin as contained in this blend could lead to permanent changes in insulin requirements. To prevent the possibility of insulin overdose, diabetic should make their physician aware of the dietary change. (*See also ENVIRONMENTAL POLLUTION*)

HAWTHORN BERRY and **CAYENNE**, in the carefully measured amounts found in this blend, will slowly eat away cholesterol deposits and provide relief from concurrent hypertension. Cayenne helps regulate cholesterol and lipid levels. (**7**). Tests a few years ago in my lab showed that serum cholesterol levels in rats maintained on a carefully controlled diet that contained 2 grams/day powdered Hawthorn berries fell anywhere from 10% to 18% over a 2 month period (**8**). One important reason for including these herbs in this blend is to provide nutritive support to the heart and circulatory system.

FENUGREEK SEED, according to European research, may be a good agent for reducing serum cholesterol (**9**). And, like Pectin, Fenugreek seeds may be an important remedy for diabetes. Fenugreek seeds contain a certain portion of mucilaginous fiber with high viscosity. The herb may affect cholesterol levels in the same fashion as Pectin. Fenugreek also contains saponins. The saponin-containing plant fibers could inhibit the intestinal absorption of cholesterol much as Alfalfa saponins do, i.e., by adsorbing bile acids and increasing the loss of bile acids by fecal excretion, which then leads to an increased conversion of cholesterol into bile acids by the liver. (*See also FEMALE TONIC; STOMACH/INTESTINAL*)

PLANTAIN SEED contains mucilage in its outer epidermis and swells when it gets wet. This property makes these seeds a natural candidate for the control of cholesterol levels. Along these lines, Plantain has been shown by scientists in Italy, Russia and other countries to reduce the intestinal absorption of lipids and cholesterol (**10**). The consensus of opinion is that the seeds and leaves act by reducing the intestinal absorption of bile acids. Cholesterol levels may also be lowered in persons that use the herb as an appetite suppressant. (*See also WEIGHT LOSS; BONE-FLESH-CARTILAGE; RESPIRATORY AILMENTS; VAGINAL YEAST INFECTION*)

BLACK COHOSH has a tonic action on the heart and circulation. It has been experimentally proven to reduce hypertension (**36**). The plant exhibits a variety of other physiological properties that are only vaguely related to each other. We desparately need more research to clarify the behavior of this herb. (*See also HIGH BLOOD PRESSURE; FEMALE TONIC; NERVOUS TENSION*)

OTHER NUTRIENTS

VITAMINS
Vitamin B Complex
Vitamin C 1,000-3,000 mg
Vitamin E 200-600 I.U.
Bioflavonoids 100-300 mg
Inositol 1,000 mg
Choline 1,000 mg
Niacinamide 100 mg
  Calcium/Magnesium
  Phosphorous
  Potassium
  Zinc

MINERALS
  GLA
  Essential Fatty Acid
  Cod Liver Oil
  Walnut Oil
  Lecithin
  Brewer's Yeast

REFERENCES

1. Lin, T.M., Kim, K.S., Karvinen, E. & Ivy, A.C. "Effect of dietary pectin, 'protopectin' and gum arabic on cholesterol excretion in rats." **American Journal of Physiology**, 188(1), 66-70, 1957.
2. Kay, R.M. & Truswell, A.S. "Effect of citrus pectin on blood lipids and fecal steroid excretion in man." **American Journal of Clinical Nutrition**, 30, 171-175, 1977.
3. Leveille, G.A. & Sauberlich, H.E. "Mechanism of the cholesterol-depressing effect of pectin in the cholesterol-fed rat." **Journal of Nutrition**, 88, 209-217, 1966.
4. Heaton, K. in **Refined carbohydrate Foods and Disease.**" Burkett, D.P. & Trowell, H.C., eds. Academic Press, London, 1975., p. 173.
5. Sharma, R.V., Sharma, S.C. & Prasad, Y. "Effect of pectin on carbohydrate and fat metabolism." **Indian Journal of Medical Research**, 76, 771-775, 1982.
6. Burkitt, D.P., Walker, A.R.P, & Painter, N.S. "Dietary fiber and diseases." **Journal of the American Medical Association**, 229, 1068-1074, 1974.
7. Sambaiah, K & Satyanarayana, N. "Hypocholesterolemic effect of red pepper & capsaicin." **Indian Journal of Experimental Biology**, 18, 898-899, 1980.
8. Mowrey, D.B. Unpublished data accumulated from June, 1978 to August, 1978 at the Nebo Institute for Herbal Sciences, Spanish Fork, Utah.
9. Valette, G., Sauvaire, Y., Baccou, J.-C., & Ribes, G. "Hypocholesterolaemic effect of fenugreek seeds in dogs." **Atherosclerosis**, 50, 105-111, 1984.
10. Maksiutina, N.P., Nikitina, N.I., Lipkan, G.N., Gorin, A.G. & Voitenko, I.N. "Chemical composition and hypocholesterolemic action of some drugs from plantago major leaves." **Famatsevtychnyi Zhurnal**, 4, 56-61, 1978.
11. Salerno **Minerva Otorinolaringologica**, 5,12, 1955.

CIRCULATION

HERBS: CAYENNE (*Capsicum annum*), **Kelp** (*Saminaria, Macrocystis, Ascophyllum*), **Gentian root** (*Gentiana lutea*), **Ginger root** (*Zingiber officinale*), **Blue Vervain** (*Verbena hastata*).

Form: Capsule.

PURPOSE: Blood. To stimulate circulation.

Other Applications: Frostbite, hypothermia, varicose veins, colds, flu, fevers, sore throat, indigestion, heartburn.

USE: 1. Poor Circulation: 2-4 caps/day.
    2. Infectious Ailments: 4-6 caps/day. Use with blends for FEVERS & INFECTIONS, and INFLUENZA:
    3. Hypothermia: 2 caps/hour. 4. Indigestion: 2 caps every 2-3 hours.
    5. To supplement blend for HEART: 2-3 caps/day.
    6. To supplement blend for HIGH BLOOD PRESSURE: 2-3 caps/day.

Contraindications: None. Do not exceed recommended use.

It is vital to all of the body's cells that they receive an adequate supply of oxygen and nutrients. Likewise, carbon dioxide and wastes must be removed. Many factors can reduce the blood's ability to deliver the goods and take away the wastes, including injuries and diseases. Under such conditions, the circulation can use a boost from external sources. Use this blend when you have a cold, or when you're cold, or if you have generally poor circulation. Use it to supplement various other blends as noted above. Under normal circumstances, please adhere to the suggested dosage. Only in case of hypothermia, bad colds, and/or severe fevers should greater quantities be consumed.

CAYENNE pepper will get your blood moving posthaste, especially in the gustatory regions. Other foods ingested along with Cayenne will be assimilated faster and more easily. The research data to support this fact is voluminous (e.g. **1-2**). One suggested explanation for this effect is that the herb releases endogenous gastric secretagogues which increase both tissue perfusion by blood and secretory activity (**1**). A little goes a long way, so don't overdo it. Remember, Nature made the stuff hot and pungent for a reason. If you can't swallow too much outside of a capsule, don't swallow too much inside of a capsule either. *(See also BLOOD PURIFICATION; HIGH BLOOD PRESSURE; FATIGUE)*

GINGER ROOT will stimulate circulation in the G.I. tract and other parts of the body, and will help the body digest and the blood assimilate the Cayenne. Ginger root has a powerful positive stimulating effect on muscular contractions of the atria (**3**); this effect should increase overall circulation. It has also been shown experimentally that Ginger root stimulates the vasomotor and respiratory centers of the central nervous system. as well as the heart (**4**). Ginger root also helps reduce serum cholesterol levels, an effect that would promote long term circulatory improvement (**5**). Finally, in a very recent test-tube study, another mechanism by which Ginger root may improve circulation was discovered. In that study, a water extract of Ginger root significantly reduced platelet aggregation (the tendency of blood cells to stick together or clot) (**6**). Agents found to possess this property are generally beneficial to the circulation. *(See also BLOOD SUGAR; FATIGUE; STOMACH/INTESTINAL; DIGESTION; LAXATIVE; NAUSEA; NERVOUS TENSION)*

GENTIAN ROOT is invaluable to the body's circulation and overall health by bolstering its ability to digest and assimilate food. In good health or bad, it increases absorption, assimilation and resorption. The effect of Gentian on the vascular system is to help insure that the abdominal organs receive a rich supply of blood. It has also been found that Gentian root increases the sensitivity of many glands and organs to the effect of adrenalin--the endogenous hormone that is secreted when the body needs quick energy (**7**). *(See also STOMACH/INTESTINAL; DIABETES; NERVES & GLANDS)*

KELP possesses cardiotonic principles of its own. In one study, it was found that Kelp increases contractile force in the atria (much like Ginger root as noted above) (**8**). In another study, two cardiac principles were isolated from Laminaria that stimulated the hearts of frogs (**9**). In addition, Kelp adds that measure of nutritive support that the body needs to maintain proper health. It helps offset the effects of stress, protects against sickness, aids digestion and respiration, and generally promotes well-being. *(See also FEVERS & INFECTIONS; WEIGHT LOSS; FATIGUE; THYROID; DIABETES; ENVIRONMENTAL POLLUTION; MENTAL ALERTNESS/SENILITY; PAIN; INFERTILITY; HEART; BLOOD PURIFICATION/DETOXIFICATION)*

BLUE VERVAIN is valued by many herbalists as an agent that will help to rectify poor circulation problems (**10**). But among its many uses, this is perhaps its most obscure, a practice cherished by those who use it, but ignored by others. Extrapolating from its proven parasympathetic properties (**11**), it should have a normalizing or stabilizing effect on the circulation. *(See also NERVES & GLANDS; FEVERS & INFECTIONS)*

OTHER NUTRIENTS

VITAMINS
(Daily requirements unless otherwise noted)
    Vitamin A *25,000 I.U. daily*
    Vitamin B-1 *25 mg*
    Vitamin B-2 *25 mg*
    Vitamin B-6 *25 mg*
    Vitamin B-12 *25 mcg*
    Vitamin C *1,000 mg*
    Vitamin D *200-400 I.U.*
    Vitamin E *200-500 I.U.*
    Pantothenic Acid *100 mg*
    PABA *15 mg*

MINERALS
    Calcium/Magnesium
    Potassium
    Iodine
    Zinc

REFERENCES

1. Limlomwongse, L., Chaitauchawong, C. & Tongyai, S. "Effect of capsaicin on gastric acid secretion and mucosal blood flow in the rat." **Journal of Nutrition**, 109, 773-777, 1979.
2. Kolatat, T. & Chungcharcon, D. "The effect of capsaicin on smooth muscle and blood flow of the stomach and the intestine." **Siriraj Hospital Gazette**, 24, 1405-1418, 1972.
3. Masada, Y., Inoue, T., Hashimoto, K., Fujioka, M. & Uchino, C. "Studies on the constituents of ginger (Zingiber officinale) by GC-MS." **Yakugaku Zasshi**, 94(6), 735-738, 1974.
4. Ally, M.M. "The pharmacological action of zingiber officinale." **Proceedings of the Pan Indian Ocean Scientific Congress, 4th, Karachi, Pakistan**, Section G, 11-12, 1960.
5. Gujral, S., Bhumka, H. & Swaroop, M. "Effect of ginger (Zingiber officinale roscoe) oleoresin on serum and hepatic cholesterol levels in cholesterol fed rats." **Nutrition Reports International**, 17(2), 183-189, 1978.
6. Srivastava, K.C. "Effects of aqueous extracts of onion, garlic and ginger on platelet aggregation and metabolism of arachidonic acid in the blood vascular system." **Prostaglandins Leukotrienes and Medicine**, 13, 227-235, 1984.
7. Deininger, R. "Amarum—bittere arznei." **Krankenpflege**, 29(3), 99-100, 1975.
8. Searl, P.B., Norton, T.R., & Lum B.K.B. "Study of a cardiotonic fraction from an extract of the seaweed *Undaria pinnatifida*." **Proceedings of the Western Pharmacology Society**, 24, 63-65, 1981.
9. Kosuge, T., Nukaya, H., Yamamotoa, T. & Tsuji, K. "Isolation and identification of cardiac principles from laminaria." **Yakugaku Zasshi**, 103(6), 683-685, 1983.
10. Hutchens, A.R. **Indian Herbalogy of North America**, Merco, Ontario, Canada, 1973.
11. Thomson, W.R. **Herbs that Heal**, Charles Scribner's Sons, New York, 1976, pp.156-157.

DETOXIFY/NURTURE

HERBS: **RED CLOVER** (*Trifolium pratense*), **CHAPARRAL** (*Larrea divaricata*), **Licorice root** (*Glycyrrhiza glabra*), **Oregon Grape root** (*Mahonia aquifolium*), **Stillingia** (*Stillingia sylvatica*), **Burdock root** (*Arctium lappa*), **Cascara Sagrada bark** (*Rhamnus purshiana*), **Sarsaparilla root** (*smilax officinalis*), **Prickly Ash bark** (*Zanthoxylum americanum*), **Buckthorn bark** (*Rhamnus frangula*), & **Kelp** (*Laminaria, Macrocystis, Ascophyllum*).

Form: Capsule, Tea

PURPOSE: Degenerative disorders: a nutritive supplement.

Other Applications: Arthritis, post-surgery trauma, neural degeneration, senility, Addison's disease.

USE: 1. 3 capsules, 3 to 4 times per day, with plenty of liquid.

2. To supplement the BLOOD PURIFICATION Blend: 1-2 capsules, 3 times per day.

3. To supplement the FEVERS & INFECTIONS Blend: 2 capsules, twice per day.

Contraindications: None. Chaparral, though sometimes called creosote bush, contains **no** creosote.

The purpose of this blend is provide nutritive and therapeutic support to the body during the course of, and during recuperation from, any debilitating condition, be it arthritis or appendicitis, major surgery or cancer, pneumonia or polio. These herbs provide a comprehensive cleansing and detoxification program including nutrition, stimulation, rejuvenation, and remedy. The combined action action of several of these herbs is even believed by some to cure cancer, though proof of that theory has never been satisfactorily shown.

RED CLOVER has been used in America for over 100 years to treat and prevent cancer, and as a sedataive for whoooping cough (2). In Europe it is used as a diuretic to treat gout, and as an expectorant. Red Clover has shown some estrogenic activity (4). Because of its high content of several important nutrients, including vitamins and minerals, Red Clover has become a dependable nutritive supplement in all forms of degenerative disease. Antibiotic tests on Red Clover have shown it to possess activity against several bacteria, the most significant of which is the pathogen that causes tuberculosis (6).

CHAPARRAL is undoubtedly beneficial for some people with certain types of cancer in certain stages of development, but it is not clear who may benefit, which cancers are most susceptible or at which stage of cancer development the herb is most effective (7). It has been repeatedly shown that NDGA (nordihydroguaiaretic acid), the purported active principle in Chaparral, is posionous to some kinds of cancer cells while not affecting normal cells (8, 9-10). *(See also SKIN DISORDERS; BONE-FLESH -CARTILAGE; ARTHRITIS)*

LICORICE ROOT is one of the great detoxifiers in nature. In China, Licorice root is known as "The Great Detoxifier." A group of Russian researchers have found that Licorice root inhibits the growth of certain tumors (sarcoma-45 and Ehrlich ascites cells) (11). Another recent study found that the herb actually stimulates the production of interferon, that critical chemical in the immune system that could be the key to preventing and treating many immune-response deficiency diseases (12).

OREGON GRAPE ROOT has a direct action on the skin. Therein it behaves unlike any other herb known. It is used to restore the skin to a smooth, clear condition following any kind of skin disease or other illness that may have dried out the skin or produced sores. Oregon Grape is also a good source of berberine which is one of the active principles in Goldenseal. In fact, the findings relating to Goldenseal, as discussed in other chapters, should apply to Oregon Grape as well. Oregon Grape has a proven strong bacteriacidal effect (13).

STILLINGIA ROOT is a North American plant that became **the** alterative of choice the last century. It was hailed by many physicians as the best treatment for syphilis known. Gradually, its other properties were explored and clinically substantiated; the final result was its acceptance as a treatment for tuberculosis and cancer, as well as all other conditions for which an alterative could be recommended (2-3,14). *(See also BLOOD PURIFICATION/DETOXIFICATION; SKIN DISORDERS.)*

BURDOCK ROOT is another classic blood purifier, or alterative. It is also diuretic and diaphoretic. So, in three different ways it helps cleanse the body of toxins and wastes, especially those that accumulate during illness. These three mechanisms are further enhanced by the herb's proven restorative effects on the liver and gallbladder (15). Antibiotic, antifungal and antitumor principles combine in this herb to provide great deal of potential value in the prevention and remedy of, and recuperation from, disease. *(See also BONE-FLESH-CARTILAGE; BLOOD PURIFICATION/DETOXIFICATION; SKIN DISORDERS)*

CASCARA SAGRADA is the primary laxative in this blend. It helps remove consolidated, bacteria-laden waste matter from the large intestine during periods of illness. Cascara does not produce griping, cramping, diarrhea or constipative rebound, and is especially well suited for the elderly (16). Several therapeutic properties, not commonly known, have been attributed to Cascara, including potent antibacterial properties (16-17). Liver diseases and leukemia have been prevented, treated, or cured by Cascara constituents (18-19). *(See also LAXATIVE; LIVER DISORDERS)*

SARSAPARILLA is used in the United States, China and other disparate countries for about the same purposes: rheumatism, arthritis, skin disease, venereal disease, fevers, digestive disorders and as a general tonic. One Chinese clinical study found a 90% degree of effectiveness against primary syphilis (5). And a couple of studies have verified the presence of antibiotic principles (6, 20). Sarsaparilla's primary purpose in this blend is to tone up the body and provide nutritive and therapeutic support for convalescent patient. *(See also BLOOD PURIFICATION/DETOXIFICATION; INFERTILITY; ARTHRITIS; WHOLE BODY)*

PRICKLY ASH BARK earned itself an incredible reputation in 1849-1850, for remedying and outbreak of Asiatic Cholera. It was also a main ingredient in a very popular compound used to treat syphilis, and was chosen for inclusion in Hoxey's famous cancer cure. Speaking of typhoid pneumonia and typhus fever, one 19th century physician wrote, "I am compelled to say that I consider the tincture of Prickly Ash berries superior to any other form of medication." (14, p. 127). Prickly Ash has been used extensively to remedy all kinds of debilitating conditions. Merck reports that asarinin, one of the lignans in Prickly Ash, has antituberular properties (21).

BUCKTHORN BARK was a part of the famous Hoxey cancer cure. Support for this claim is found in a study in which certain Buckthorn preparations showed significant inhibition of P-388 lymphocytic leukemia in mice (22). The major constituents of Buckthorn are anthraquinone glycosides, which are mildly laxative in nature. Buckthorn is the mildest anthraquinone-containing herb, just ahead of Cascara (1, 23). The anthraquinones help rid the body of accumulations of toxic waste.

KELP supplies an incredible number of nutrients and possesses numerous medicinal properties of its own. Note especially its anti-cancer, anti-rheumatic, anti-inflammatory, hypotensive and fibrous qualities. For details on these, the reader is referred to several other blends: *(See also*

OTHER NUTRIENTS

VITAMINS
(Daily requirements unless otherwise noted)

Vitamin A 50,000 I.U.	Vitamin C 3,000-5,000 mg
Vitamin B Complex	Vitamin D 800 I.U.
Vitamin B1 25-100 mg	Vitamin E 400-600 I.U.
Vitamin B2 25-100 mg	Niacinamide 100 mg
Vitamin B6 25-100 mg	PABA 30 mg
Vitamin B12 150 mcg	Pantothenic acid 200mg

MINERALS
Calcium/Magnesium
Phosphorous
Zinc
Iodine

MISCELLANEOUS
HCl

REFERENCES

1. List, P.H. & Hoerhammer, L. **Hagers Handbuch der Pharmazeutischen Praxis.** Volumes 2-5, Springer-Verlag, Berlin.
2. Ellingwood, F. **American Materia Medica, Therapeutics and Pharmacognosy.** Eclectic Medical Publications, Portland, Oregon, 1983.
3. Felter, H. W. **The Eclectic Materia Medica, Pharmacology and Therapeutics.** Eclectic Medical Publications, Portland, Oregon, 1983 (first published 1922).
4. Schultz, G. "Content of estrogenic isoflavones in red clover (trifilium pratense) cultivated in sand with different mineral supplies." **Deutsche Tieraerztliche Wochenschrift**, 74(5), 118-120, 1967.
5. Leung, A.Y. **Encyclopedia of Common Natural Ingredients.** New York, 1980.
6. Fitzpatrick, F.K. "Plant substances active against mycobacterium tuberculosis." **Antibiotics and Chemotherapy**, 4(5), 528-536, 1954.
7. Smart, C.R., Hogle, H.H., Vogel, H., Broom, A.D. & Bartholomew, D. "Clinical experience with nordihydroguaiaretic acid—Chaparral (sic) tea in the treatment of cancer." **Rocky Mountain Medical Journal**, November, 1970, 39-43.
8. Sporn, A. & Schobesch, O. "Toxicity of nordihydroquaiaretic acid." **Igiena** (Bucharest), 15(12), 725-726, 1966.
9. Schwarz, M., Peres, G., Kunz, W. et al "On the role of superoxide anion radicals in skin tumor promotion." **Carcinogenesis**, 5(12), 1663-1670, 1984.

10. Carine, K., & Hudig, D. "Assessment of a role for phospholipase A2 and arachidonic acid metabolism in human lymphocyte natural cytotoxicity." **Cellular Immunology**, 87(1), 270-283, 1984.

11. Shvarev, I.F. Konovalova, N.K. & Putilova, G.I. "Effect of triterpenoid compounds from glycyrrhiza glabra on experimental tumors." **Voprosy Izucheniya Ispol'zovaniy. Solodki v SSSR, Akademi Nauk SSSR**, 167-170, 1966.

12. Abe, N., Eina, T. & Ishida, N. "Interferon induction by glycyrrhizin and glycyrrhetinic acid in mice." **Micorobiology and Immunology**, 26(6), 535-539, 1982.

13. Kowalewski, Z., Kedzia, W. & Mirska, I. "Effect of berberine sulfate on staphylococci." **Archives of Immunology and Experimental Therapeutics**, 20(3), 353-360, 1972.

14. Millspaugh, C. F. **American Medicinal Plants**. Dover Publications, Inc. New York, 1974 (first published 1892).

15. Chabrol, E. & Charonnat, R. "Therapeutic agents in bile secretion." **Ann. Med.**, 37, 131-142, 1935.

16. Marchesi, M., Marcato, M. & Silvestrini, C. "A laxative mixture in the therapy of constipation in aged patients." **Giornale di Clinica Medica**,(Bologna) 63, 850-863, 1982.

17. Anton, R. & Duquenois, P. "Cassia marilandica in therapy with medicinal plants." **Quarterly Journal of Crude Drug Research**, 9(4), 1469-1472, 1969.

18. Cudlin, J., Blumauerova, M. Steinerova, N., Mateju, J. & Zalabak, V. "Biological activity of hydroxyanthraquinones and their glucosides toward microorganisms." **Folia Microbiologica (Prague)**, 21(1), 54-57, 1976.

19. Chen, C.H., Cheng, W.F., Su, H.L., et. al. "Studies on chinese rhubarb. I. Preliminary study on the antibacterial activity of anthraquinone derivatives of chinese rhubarb (rheum palmatum)." **Acta Pharmaceutica Sinica (Yao Hsueh Hsueh Pao)**, 9, 757-762, 1962.

20. D'Amico, M.L. "Ricerche sulla presenza di sostanze ad azione antibiotica nelle piante superiori." **Fitoterapia**, 21(1), 77-79, 1950.

21. **The Merck Index. An Encyclopedia of Chemicals and Drugs.** 9th ed., 1976, Merck. Rahway, NJ.

22. Kupchan, S.M. & Karim, A. "Tumor inhibitors 114: Aloe emodin: antileukemic principle isolated from Rhamnus frangula L." **Lloydia**, 39, 223-224, 1976.

23. Youngken, H.W. **Textbook of Pharmacognosy**, 5th ed. Blakiston, Philadelphia, PA, 1943.

DIABETES

HERBS: UVA-URSI (*Arctostaphylos uva-ursi*), **DANDELION** root (*Taraxacum officinale*), **Parsley** (*Petroselinum sativum*), **Gentian root** (*Gentiana lutea*), **Huckleberry leaves** (*Vaccinum myrtillus*), **Raspberry leaves** (*Rubus idaeus*), **Buchu leaves** (*Barosma crenata*), **Saw Palmetto berries** (*Serenoa repens-sabal*), **Kelp** (*Laminara, Macrocystes, Ascophyllum*), & **Bladderwrack** (*Fucus vesiculosus*).

Form: Capsule, Tea

PURPOSE: Promotes the body's ability to reduce high blood sugar (hyperglycemia); promotes glandular health and function.

Other Applications: Diuretic.

USE: 1. For Hyperglycemia: 3 caps, 3 times per day.
2. For Glandular Health: 2-4 caps per day.
3. Use 2-4 caps per day of the NERVE & GLAND TONIC Blend for added benefit to glands.
4. If used with the DIURETIC Blend, use 2-4 capsules per day of each.

Contraindications: 1. Do not use if nephritis exists. 2. Should not be used by hypoglycemics. 3. Persons who use diuretics often, who are generally rundown, or have a known potassium deficiency, should use caution when using any diuretic product, and should definitely take potassium supplements. 4. Frequent consultation with your physician is recommended to adjust insulin-intake requirements, as this blend may significantly reduce necessary insulin supplementation.

Diabetes is a defect in carbohydrate metabolism that results from insufficient pancreatic insulin production. The diabetic often requires a daily insulin injection so that he can consume moderate amounts of carbohydrate. Any dietary treatment that can reduce or eliminate the need for insulin injections will increase the diabetic's ability to avoid serious symptoms This blend is about the best adjunctive aid Mother Nature can supply, but it is not meant to supplant qualified medical care. It will provide sound functional support to the physiological systems involved, and may depress the blood sugar level in any given individual (and should therefore not be used by hypoglycemics).

UVA URSI helps relieve pain from bladder stones and gravel, relieves cystitis, nephritis and kidney stones (**1**). Early in American history, Uva-ursi was felt to be of great benefit in numerous ailments, as an astringent and anti-scorbutic, and was used as food by Indians and the English (**2**). Shortly thereafter, other American researchers found that Uva-ursi was effective against nephritis and kidney stones, and possessed all around tonic properties (**3**). Today, the herb is used as a tonic and specific in cases involving weakened liver, kidneys and other glands. *(See also DIURETIC; MENSTRUATION)*

DANDELION ROOT exhibits hypoglycemic effects in experimental animals (**5**). Dandelion's beneficial effects on liver complaints have been documented by both Asian practitioners (**6**) and American physicians (**4**). It stimulates bile production and helps the body get rid of excess water produced by the diseased liver. Dandelion extracts are said to also benefit the spleen and improve the health of the pancreas. *(See also LIVER DISORDERS; NERVES & GLANDS; BLOOD PURIFICATION/DETOXIFICATION; SKIN)*

PARSLEY is commonly used to treat jaundice and gallstones. Its influences on the liver have not been experimentally investigated. But clinical physicians, over the past 100 years or so, have widely claimed that the herb is very effective in remedying liver diseases (**7**). *(See also PROSTATE; DIURETIC; BONE-FLESH-CARTILAGE)*

GENTIAN ROOT has been used by both Western and Eastern societies as a potent bitter. Its focus of activity is on those glands and organs involved in digestion, such as the gallbladder and pancreas, with secondary affects on other organs such as the liver and kidneys. It has been found experimentally to promote the secretion of bile (**8**). The diabetic or pre-diabetic will experience increased pancreatic health when the herb is used as a tonic. Gentian, today, is regarded as one of the premier herbs to use when any gland of the body is malfunctioning or severely stressed. *(See also NERVES & GLANDS; CIRCULATION; STOMACH/INTESTINAL; THYROID)*

HUCKLEBERRY LEAF is used by many naturopathic physicians to treat sugar diabetes, and ailments of the kidneys and gallbladder (**9**). This is not surprising since the Huckleberry is a close cousin, if not brother, to Uva-ursi, its leaves containing very similar compounds as that plant. The active principle is neomyrtilicine. The herb is one of the best for mild diabetes; and may be especially beneficial for use in "senile" diabetes.

RASPBERRY LEAF is primarily used for diarrhea and for problems associated with female biology, but is used frequently in folk medicine to relieve urethral and kidney irritation (**10**). There is some experimental support for using Raspberry leaf to treat diabetes: the leaf has a proven hypoglycemic action. (**11**). *(See also EYES; MENSTRUATION; FEMALE TONIC)*

BUCHU LEAF is aromatic and carminative. It helps to relieve irritation of the bladder, urethra and kidneys (**7**). *(See also PROSTATE; DIURETIC; VAGINAL YEAST INFECTION)*

SAW PALMETTO BERRY is effectively used for nutritional support of all bodily systems. It helps build new tissue and restore function. Its inclusion in this blend is precisely for the reason that diabetes and other diseases of the glands and organs require the kind of nutritive and chemical support that these berries provide. *(See also THYROID; INFERTILITY; RESPIRATORY AILMENTS; FEMALE TONIC; PROSTATE; NERVES & GLANDS; DIGESTION)*

KELP, due to its high iodine content, is a necessary inclusion in any product that purports to help the glands (esp. thyroid and liver). Kelp contains a sugar that is mildly sweet yet does not raise blood sugar levels. It is thought that Kelp may someday become a source for a sweetening agent that diabetics can use. *(See also FEVERS & INFECTIONS; WEIGHT LOSS; FATIGUE; BLOOD PURIFICATION/DETOXIFICATION; HEART; INFERTILITY; PAIN; MENTAL ALERTNESS/SENILITY; ENVIRONMENTAL POLLUTION; THYROID; CIRCULATION)*

BLADDERWRACK, another product of the sea, has been effective against nephritis, bladder inflammation, cardiac degeneration, obesity, thyroid problems, and menstrual problems (**12**).

OTHER NUTRIENTS

VITAMINS
(Daily requirements unless otherwise noted)

Vitamin A 25,000 I.U.	Vitamin D 400 I.U.
Vitamin B1 25-50 mg	Vitamin E 200-600 I.U.
Vitamin B2 25-50 mg	Niacinamide 100 mg
Vitamin B6 25-100 mg	Pantothenic Acid 50 mg
Vitamin B12 50-100 mg	Biotin
Vitamin C 1,000-3,000 mg	

MINERALS	MISCELLANEOUS
Potassium	Water
Zinc	Essential Fatty Acids
Chromium	Complex Carbohydrate
Manganese	Lecithin
Calcium/Magnesium	Yeast
	Protein

REFERENCES

1. Lust, J. **The Herb Book**. 1974. Benedict Lust. Sini Valley, Calif.

2. Josselyn, J. "New England's Rarities Discovered, in Birds, Beasts, Fishes, Serpents, and Plants of that Country", **Archaeologica Americana, Transactions and Collections of the American Antiquarian Society**. Boston, 1860, Vol IV,105-238.

3. Barton, B.S. **Collections for an Essay towards a Materia Medica of the United States**. 3rd Ed., with additions. Philadelphia, printed for Edward Earle and Co., 1810.

4. Clapp, A. "Report on Medical Botany...A synopsis, of systematic catalogue of the indigenous and naturalized, flowering and filicoid...medicinal plants of the United States..." **Transactions of the American Medical Association**, Vol V, 1852, Philadelphia.

5. Farnsworth, N.R. & Segelman, A.B. "Hypoglycemic plants" Tile Till. 1971, 57, 52-55.

6. Li Shih-chen, **Chinese Medicinal Herbs**. Translated by F. Porter Smith and G.A. Stuart. Georgetown Press, San Francisco, 1973.

7. Culbreth, D.M.R. **A Manual of Materia Medica and Pharmacology**, Philadelphia, 1927.

8. Sadritdinov, F. "Comparative study of the antiinflammatory properties of alkaloids from gentiana plants." **Farmakologia Alkaloidov Serdechnykh Glikozidov**, 146-148, 1971.

9. Turova, M.A. **Lekarstvennye Sredstava Iz Rastenyi** (Medical-Herbal Preparations). Publisher: Medicinskaya Literatura, Moscow, 1962.

10. Leek, S. **Herbs, Medicine & Mysticism**. Chicago. Henry Regnery Co. 1975.

11. **Planta Medica**. 11, 159, 1963.

12. Felter, H.W. **The Eclectic Materia Medica, Pharmacology and Therapeutics**. Eclectic Medical Pubs, Portland, Oregon, 1983 (first published, 1922).

DIGESTION

HERBS: PAPAYA leaves (*Carica papaya*), PEPPERMINT leaves (*Mentha piperita*), **Ginger root** (*Zingiber officinalez*), *Catnip* (*Nepeta cataria*), **Fennel seed** (*Foeniculum vulgare*), & **Saw Palmetto berries** (*Serenoa repens-sabal*).

Form: Capsule, Tea, Poultice

PURPOSE: Digestive aid; Intestinal gas (flatulence); Enteritis; Colic; Heartburn.

Other Applications: Ulcers; Worms.

USE: 1. For indigestion, use 2 caps with each meal.

2. To supplement the STOMACH/INTESTINAL Blend: 2 caps of each blend, with meals.

3. To supplement the PARASITES & WORMS Blend: 1-2 caps/day.

Contraindications: None.

Digestion is an amazingly complex process that involves and depends upon the proper functioning of a series of valves, gates, enzyme secreting plants, properly buffered processing facilities, microscopic filtration, absorption, resorption, motoric churning, pumping and crunching. This herbal blend focuses mainly on the chemical processes involved, though some tonic strengthening of the motoric functions is also involved. Indigestion (dyspepsia) is both a physiological state and a feeling. The state is one of faulty digestion. The feeling is one of discomfort, being "stuffed", pain, cramps, heartburn, gas and nausea. Indigestion may often be a symptom of a greater problem, in which case the advice of a physician should be obtained. This blend of herbs will help reduce digestive and intestinal complaints in two distinct ways. First it enhances digestion itself. Second, it remedies the various side-effects of poor digestion: flatulent gas, colic, heartburn, etc. Keep this blend handy and use it frequently. Don't forget to also use the LIVER PROBLEMS blend.

PAPAYA LEAF contains the powerful proteolytic enzymes papain and chymopapain, which digest proteins, small peptides, amides and esters. Their activity extends also to carbohydrate and fat. They are more effective than naturally occurring proteases like pepsin and trypsin. Since many stomach ailments are the direct result of indigestion, Papaya may help prevent and remedy these by increasing digestive processes. The digestive properties of papain are well established (e.g. **1-3**). *(See also STOMACH/INTESTINAL; MENSTRUATION)*

PEPPERMINT LEAF contains volatile oils and other constituents that absorb intestinal gas, calm upset stomach, inhibit diarrhea as well as constipation, aid digestion, eliminate heartburn, and prevent and remedy childhood colic. Peppermint is probably the best known remedy for stomach problems. It is used for both chronic and acute indigestion, gastritis and enteritis, acting in two distinct ways to remedy these problems. First, its essential oils enhance digestive activity by stimulating contractile activity in the gallbladder and by encouraging the secretion of bile (**4**). Secondly, Peppermint leaf oils normalize gastrointestinal activity, removing flaccidity and reducing cramps (**5**). *(See also MENTAL ALERTNESS/SENILITY; FATIGUE)*

GINGER ROOT's primary activity is described elsewhere in this book (see STOMACH/INTESTINAL, CIRCULATION, NAUSEA). Of great importance here are these findings: 1) Ginger root contains a digestive enzyme, zingibain, whose effectiveness even exceeds that of papain (**6**); 2) the herb stimulates the flow of saliva and increases dramatically the concentration of digestive enzyme (amylase) in the saliva (**7**); 3) it activates peristalsis and increases intestinal muscle tone (**7**). The ability of Ginger root to clear up gas, flatulence, indigestion, stomachache and other stomach problems has been repeatedly confirmed in my own experimental investigations (**8**). *(See also FATIGUE; NERVOUS TENSION; LOW BLOOD SUGAR; NAUSEA; CIRCULATION; LAXATIVE; STOMACH/INTESTINAL)*

CATNIP, often called Catmint, acts in much the same manner as Peppermint. It is a soothing carminative to the gastrointestinal tract, a mild tonic, and a favorite tea for young children. North American Indians used the tea for childhood colic, while Europeans used it for similar complaints as well as colds and bronchial infections. Used before meals, it stimulates appetite; after meals it stimulates digestion. Catnip is sometimes called "Nature's Alka Seltzer," though that term aptly describes the whole Mint family.

FENNEL SEEDS contain aromatic or essential oils that are very similar in structure and activity to those of Catnip and Peppermint (**9**). Fennel appears to be equally effective in children and adults. It is especially effective against flatulence in adults. Fennel was official in the U.S. Pharmacopoeia for many years and is still official in over a dozen major foreign pharmacopoeias worldwide. *(See also WEIGHT LOSS)*

SAW PALMETTO BERRY is included in this blend on the basis of there commendations and celebrations of people who have used it, and doctors who have prescribed it, to stimulate the appetite, improve digestion and increase assimilation. Their enthusiasm has been justified by at least one corroborating study in which young albino rats, to whose daily feed crushed Saw Palmetto berries were added, experienced a significantly more rapid weight gain than control litter mates (**10**). *(See also INFERTILITY; FEMALE TONIC; RESPIRATORY AILMENTS; DIABETES; PROSTATE; NERVES & GLANDS; THYROID)*

OTHER NUTRIENTS

VITAMINS
(Daily requirements unless otherwise noted)
Vitamin B Complex
Vitamin B1 *25-50 mg*
Vitamin B2 *25-50 mg*
Vitamin B6 *25-50 mg*
Folic Acid *400 mcg*
Niacinamide *100 mg*
Pantothenic Acid *50 mg*

MINERALS
Calcium/Magnesium

MISCELLANEOUS
Betain HCl
Pepsin
Pancreatin
Ox Bile
Yogurt/Acidophilus

REFERENCES

1. Yamamoto, A. in **Enzymes in Food Processing**,2nd Ed., G. Geed, ed., Academic Press, New York, 1975, p.123.

2. Arnon, R. **Methods in Enzymology**, VI 19, G.E. Perlmann and L. Lorand, eds., Academic Press, New York, 1970, p. 226.

3. Kunimatsu, D.K. & Yasunobu, K.T., in **Methods in Enzymology**, Vol 19, G.E. Perlmann and L. Lorand, eds., Academic Press, New York, 1970, p. 244.

4. List, P.H. & Hoerhammer, L. **Hagers Handbuch der Pharmazeutischen Praxis**. Volumes 2-5, Springer-Verlag, Berlin.

5. Demling, L., et. al., **Fortschritte der Medizin**, 37, 1305, 1969.

6. Thompson, E.H., Wolk, I.D. & Allen, C.E. "Ginger rhizome: a new source of proteolytic enzyme." **Journal of Food Science**, 38(4), 652-655, 1973.

7. Glatzel, H. **Deutsche. Apotheker Zeitung**, 110, 5, 1970.

8. Mowrey, D.B. Work performed between 1975-1979 on animals and in humans, some of which has been published (see references in STOMACH/INTESTINAL chapter.

9. Shipochliev, T. **Veterinarno-Meditsinski Nauki**, 5(6), 63-69, 1968.

10. Mowrey, D.B. Unpublished study, performed during routine toxicological screenings, 1978, Spanish Fork, Utah.

DIURETIC

HERBS: CORNSILK (*Stigmata maydis*), **Parsley** (*Petroselinum sativum*), **Uva-Ursi leaves** (*Arctostaphylos uva-ursi*), **Cleavers** (*Galium aparine*), **Buchu** leaves (*Barosma crenata*), **Juniper berries** (*Juniperus communis*), **Kelp** (*Laminaria, Macrocystis Ascophyllum*), **Cayenne** (*Capsicum annuum*), & **Queen-of-the-Meadow Root** (*Eupatorium purpureum*).

Form: Capsule.

PURPOSE: Diuretic; For edema and all edematous conditions; Also a treatment for urinary deficiency and infection.

Other Applications: Arthritis, For Cleanses/Detoxification, Gout

USE: 1. Acute irritation and edematous conditions: 5-8 caps/day while condition persists.
2. Urinary tract infections: 3 caps, 3 times per day.
3. Arthritis supplement: 3-4 caps/day maximum while using the ARTHRITIS Blend.
4. Cleanses & Detoxification: 5-8 caps/day; 3-4 caps/day of the SKIN DISORDERS and BLOOD PURI/DETOX Blends.
5. Obesity: 2 caps/day. Use WEIGHT LOSS Blend also.

Contraindications: 1. Do not use if nephritis exists. 2. Persons who use diuretics often, who are often rundown, or have a known potassium insufficiency should exercise caution and consider the use of supplemental potassium when using diuretics. 3. Avoid using this blend on a continuous basis. 4. Avoid high sodium foods when using this blend.

A diuretic is any substance that increases the rate of formation and secretion of urine by the kidneys. Decreased excretion of water and electrolytes by the kidneys leads to edema (increase in extracellular body fluid). Edema is treated with diuretics. There are, fortunately, literally hundreds of natural diuretics. This blend includes some of the most effective, yet mild acting, diuretic herbs available. This blend is also a potent urinary aid, affecting all forms of urinary infection, inflammation, and disease. When using diuretics you should be under a physician's care. *Note:* Ingestion of large quantities of this blend could turn the urine dark—a harmless condition.

PARSLEY, judging by its related pharmacological properties, including laxative, hypotensive and expectorant (**1-2**), probably obtains its diuretic activity by directly inhibiting salt reabsorption by body tissues. *(See also BONE-FLESH-CARTILAGE; DIABETES; PROSTATE)*

CORNSILK has been shown in recent research to be highly diuretic yet mild and non-toxic (**3**). Of course, Chinese and early eclectic physicians knew that already. Dropsical conditions are especially susceptible to the moderate diuretic principles in Cornsilk. *(See also PROSTATE)*

UVA URSI LEAF is recognized by medical authorities as diuretic, astringent and antiseptic (**5**). Arbutin, the primary active principle, has been shown to be an effective urinary disinfectant if the urine is alkaline (**6**). Uva ursi acts directly on the kidneys to achieve its diuretic effect. *(See also DIABETES; MENSTRUATION)*

CLEAVERS probably acts directly on the kidneys much like Uva-ursi. Its action is weaker and more mild, although its specific action on acute inflammation or irritation of the urinary tract is stronger than most treatments. Hypotensive principles have been isolated from Cleavers (**7**). Hypotensive activity could be important if you use this blend in a treatment probram for heart disease.

BUCHU LEAF acts directly on the kidneys and the urinary apparatus in general, increasing the fluids and solids of the urine (**8**). It is used mainly for diseases of the kidney and urinary tract, but has been applied for scores of other ailments. Its diuretic action is due to a volatile oil that promotes diuresis and imparts its recognized odor to the urine. *(See also PROSTATE; VAGINAL YEAST INFECTION)*

JUNIPER BERRY also acts directly on the kidneys, stimulating the flow of urine by raising the rate of glomerulus filtration (the process by which blood is purified and wastes filtered out) (**9**). The herb is particularly soothing to the kidneys and is therefore a valuable component of this blend. After acute nephritic illness, Juniper will return the renal epithelium to normal secretory action and normalize blood pressure (**4**). Overdoses may irritate the kidneys, but this blend is formulated to obtain the maximum benefit from Juniper berries without the risk of overdose. *(See also VAGINAL YEAST INFECTION)*

QUEEN-OF-THE-MEADOW ROOT has found widespread use In North America from the earliest years until present. Investigators of Indian medicine found that several tribes used this herb in the same manner as the whites (**10**). It is used primarily as a diuretic (for which reason it is often called gravel root), stimulant and astringent tonic, directly influencing chronic renal and cystic problems, especially where uric acid levels are high (**11**). It produces reliable urine flow in cases where the desire is there, but the product is being suppressed. *(See also ARTHRITIS)*

KELP & CAYENNE import nutritional and chemical support for this blend. They possess little diuretic action, but are included in recognition of the fact that diuretics deplete the body of several nutrients and electrolytes that these herbs can replace.

OTHER NUTRIENTS

VITAMINS

Vitamin B Complex
Vitamin B1 *25-100 mg*
Vitamin B2 *25-100 mg*
Vitamin B6 *25-100 mg*
Vitamin C *2,000-5,000mg*
Vitamin E *200-400 I.U.*

MINERALS
Potassium
Copper
Magnesium

REFERENCES

1. Opdyke, D.L.J. "Parsley seed oil." **Food and Cosmetics Toxicology** 13 (Suppl.), 897-898, 1975.
2. Kaczmarek, F., Ostrowska, B. & Szpunar, K. "Spasmolytic and diuretic activity of the more important components of petroselinum sativum." **Biuletyn Instytutu Roslin Leczniczych (Poznan),** 8, 111-117, 1962.
3. Kiangsu Institute of Modern Medicine. **Encyclopedia of Chinese Drugs.** 2 vols. Shanghai Scientific and Technical Publications. Shanghai Peoples Republic of China, 555.
4. Ellingwood, F. **American Materia Medica, Therapeutics and Pharmacognosy.** Eclectic Medical Pubs., Portland, Oregon, 1983.
5. **Martindale: The Extra Pharmacopoeia.** The Pharmaceutical Press. London. 1977.
6. List, P. H. & Hoerhammer, L. **Hagers Handbuch der Pharmazeutishcen Praxis.** Vols. 2-5, Springer-Verlag. Berlin. 1969-1976.
7. Knott, R.P. & McCutcheon, R.S. "Phytochemical investigation of a rubiaceae, galium triflorum." **Journal of Pharmaceutical Sciences,** 50(11), 963-965, 1961.
8. Claus, E.P. **Pharmacognosy.** 4th ed. Lea & Febiger. Philadelphia, Pa. 1974.
9. Racz-Kotilla, E. & Racz, G. **Farmacia,** 19, 165, 1971.
10. Mooney, J. "The Sacred Formulas of the Cherokees," **Seventh Annual Report of the Bureau of American Ethnology,** 1885-86, 301-397.
11. King, J. **The American Dispensatory.** Cincinnati, 1866.

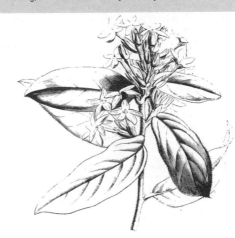

HERBS: ALGIN (*from seaweed and algae*), **Wheat bran**, **Apple pectin**, **Alfalfa** (*Medicago sativa*), & **Kelp** (*Laminaria, Macrocytes, Ascophyllum*).

Form: Capsule.

PURPOSE: To increase the body's ability to resist the effects of Environmental pollution and Heavy metal toxicity.

Other Applications: To lower serum cholesterol levels; radiation, microwave exposure; to obtain sufficient fiber (colitis, obesity, appendicitis, constipation, gallstones, etc.); vitamin A absorption, colds, flu, cancer prevention, atherosclerosis.

USE:
1. Prevention and General Purpose: 2-4 caps/day.
2. Treatment: 2 caps every 8 hours as needed.
3. Vitamin C supplementation will enhance this blend's effectiveness.

Contraindications: None. Be sure to supplement with Vitamin E (200 I.U. daily) when using any product that contains raw Alfalfa. In addition, some individuals may demonstrate a normal allergic reaction to Alfalfa. Diabetics may experience lowered insulin requirements as a result of using this blend (see CHOLESTEROL REGULATION), and should inform their physicians of this dietary change.

Illustrating the plant kingdom's ability to serve the evolving needs of humankind, this blend helps the body protect itself against the debilitating effects of a peculiarly modern problem: pollution. Though historical perspectives for herbal manipulation of this problem are irrelevant, we can rely on modern research findings that indicate it is possible to battle the effects of pollution with sound herbal methods.

ALGIN & KELP offer incredibly good protection from many kinds of modern day pollutants, carcinogens and toxins. Algin prevents living tissue from absorbing radioactive materials (**1-2**). Kelp encourages the action of dietary fiber, by supplying nutrients, and by normalizing bowel functions. Many species of Kelp have been found to possess antioxidant, anticarcinogenic, and antitoxic properties (e.g, **3-4**). Kelp may reduce the risks of poisoning from many sources of environmental pollution by providing a source of nondigestible fiber that increases fecal bulk, by reducing cholesterol levels through the inhibition of bile acid absorption (**5**), by altering the nature of fecal flora, or by a direct cytotoxic effect (**6**).

BRAN and *PECTIN* protect blood and tissue against various environmental toxins by ensuring the regular cleansing of the bowel, and by complexing with certain air and water-borne pollutants. Bran and Pectin are types of fiber. Fiber-rich diets lead to decreases in body weight, blood sugar levels, serum cholesterol and total triglycerides (**7-8**), with corresponding improvements in health. Not all dietary fibers produce the same metabolic effects. *Cellulosics* and *Hemicellulosics*, including Bran, cereals, grains, and beans, have a normalizing effect on the bowel, prevent constipation by accelerating the passage of material through the large intestine, and protect the body from disease. *Gums* including oats, guar, Irish Moss and locust beans, serve much the same purpose as the cellulosics. *Pectins*, including apples, citrus fruits, potatoes, strawberries and green beans, bind with bile acids, and decrease cholesterol levels and fat absorption. *Lignins*, plant polymers that combine with cellulose to form plant cell walls and the cementing material between them, reduce time of passage of stomach contents, bind with bile acids and lower cholesterol levels.

Pectin has the greatest effect on cholesterol levels. A few studies indicate that Bran from wheat, corn and sugar beets lowers serum cholesterol levels, but most data fail to show a significant effect in that direction (**9**). Oat bran, which is partly mucilaginous, does lower cholesterol levels substantially (**10**). Mucilaginous fiber (pectin, oat bran) rather than particulate fiber (cellulosics, most brans, lignins) is therefore responsible for decreased serum cholesterol levels. According to Soviet investigators, heavy metals, such as lead and mercury, are excreted harmlessly from the body much more efficiently when Pectin is included in the diet (**11**). Apple pectin, Rice Bran, Wheat Bran, Alfalfa fiber and Burdock root fiber, along with other sources of dietary fiber, have been shown to protect the body, and especially the gut, against the toxic effects of several common food additives (e.g., **12-13**).

ALFALFA is one the most studied plants. We know it contains many important substances, including several saponins, many sterols, flavanoids, coumarins, alkaloids, acids, vitamins, amino acids, sugars, proteins (25% by weight), minerals, trace elements and other nutrients. Alfalfa saponins inhibit increases in blood cholesterol levels by 25% when high cholesterol diets are fed to monkeys (**14**), rats (**15**), and rabbits (**16**).

Other components of Alfalfa probably enhance the action of the saponins by binding the bile acids that are necessary for cholesterol absorption. French scientists have shown that Alfalfa can reduce tissue damage caused by another modern hazard, radiotherapy (**17**). Also of interest are the effects of Vitamin K, found in high concentrations in Alfalfa. In man, dietary Vitamin K can remedy bleeding disorders which occur when the delivery of bile to the bowel is hindered, as for example in obstructive jaundice or biliary fistula (**18**). It is important to realize that Alfalfa is also fiber. As such it has been shown, along with Bran and Pectin to bind and neutralize various types of agents carcinogenic to the colon (**19**). Finally, some work suggests that Alfalfa induces activity in a complex cellular system that inactivates dietary chemical carcinogens in the liver and small intestine before they have a chance to do the body any harm. (**20**). *(See also ARTHRITIS; WHOLE BODY TONIC)*

OTHER NUTRIENTS

VITAMINS
(Daily requirements unless otherwise noted)

Vitamin A *10,000 I.U.*	Vitamin D *400 I.U.*
Vitamin B Complex	Vitamin E *400 I.U.*
Vitamin B1 *25 mg*	Choline *1,000 mg*
Vitamin B2 *25 mg*	Inositol *1,000 mg*
Vitamin B6 *25 mg*	PABA *30 mg*
Vitamin B12 *3 mcg*	Folic Acid *400 mcg*
Vitamin C *500-1,000 mg*	. Pantothenic Acid *50 mg*

MINERALS
Calcium/Magnesium
Phosphorous

MISCELLANEOUS
GLA
Essential Fatty Acid
Brewer's yeast
Yogurt/acidophilus

REFERENCES

1. Tanaka, Y., Hurlburt, A.J., Argeloff, L, Skoryna, S.C. & Stara, J.F. "Application of algal polysaccharides as in vivo binders of metal pollutant." in **Proceedings of the Seventh International Seaweed Symposium**, Wiley & Sons, New York, 1972, 602-607.

2. Humphreys, E.R. & Howells, G.R."Degradation of sodium alginate by gamma-irradiation and by oxidative-reductive depolymerization." **Carbohydrate Research**, 16(1), 65-69, 1971.

3. Hirayama, T. "Epidemiology of breast cancer with special reference to the role of diet." **Preventive Medicine**, 7, 173-195, 1978.

4. Wynder, E.L. "Dietary habits and cancer epidemiology.". **Cancer**, supplement, 43(5), 1955-1961, 1979.

5. Iritani, N. & Nogi, J. "Effect of spinach and wakame on cholesterol turnover in the rat." **Atherosclerosis**, 15, 87-92, 1972.

6. Yamamoto, I. Nagumo, T, Yagi, K. Tominaga, H. & Aoki, M. "Antitumor effect of seaweeds. 1. Antitumor effect of extracts from Sargassum and Laminaria." **Japanese Journal of Experimental Medicine**, 44(6), 543-546, 1974.

7. Albrink, M.J. "Dietary fiber, plasma insulin and obesity." **American Journal of Clinical Nutrition**, 31(10), S277S278, 1978.

8. Reiser, S. "Effect of dietary fiber on parameters of glucose tolerance in humans." In Inglett, G.E.; Falkehag, S.I.: **Dietary fibers. Chemistry and nutrition**. Academic Press, New York, 1979, p. 173.

9. van Berge-Henegouwen, G.P., Huybregts, .W., van de Werf, S., Demacker, P. & Schade, R.W. "Effect of a standardized wheat bran preparation on serum lipids in young healthy males." **American Journal of Clinical Nutrition**, 32, 794-798, 1979.

10. Anderson, J.W., Lin Chen, W. J.L. "Plant fiber. Carbohydrate and lipid metabolism." **American Journal of Clinical Nutrition**, 32(2), 346-363, 1979.

11. O.D. Livshits, "Prophylactic role of pectin-containing foods during lead poisonings." **Voprosy Pitaniya**, 28(4), 76-77, 1969. And O.G. Arkhipova & Zorina, L.A. **Professional'nye Zabolevaniya V Khimicheskoi Promyshlennosti**, 210-213, 1965.

12. Ershoff, B.H. & Thurston, E.W. "Effects of diet on amaranth (FD & C Red NO. 2) toxicity in the rat." **Journal of Nutrition**, 104, 937, 1974.

13. Ershoff, B.H. & Marshall, W.E. "Protective effects of dietary fiber in rats fed toxic doses of sodium cyclamate and polyoxyethylene sorbitan monostearate (Tween 60)." **Journal of Food Science**, 40, 357, 1975.

14. Malinow, M.R., Mclaughlin, P. & Papworth, L. "Hypocholesterolemic effect of alfalfa in cholesterol-fed monkeys." **IVth International Symposium on Atherosclerosis**, Tokyo, Japan, 1976.

15. Malinow, M.R., McLaughlin, P., Papworth, L., Stafford, C., et al. "Effect of alfalfa saponins on intestinal cholesterol absorption in rats." **American Journal of Clinical Nutrition**, 30, 2061-2067, 1977.

16. Cookson, F.B. & Federoff, S. "Quantitative relationships between administered cholesterol and alfalfa required to prevent hypercholesterolaemia in rabbits." **British Journal of Experimental Pathology**, 49, 348-355, 1968.

17. De Froment, P. "Unsaponifiable substance from alfalfa for pharmaceuticals and cosmetic use." **French Patent 2,187,328**, 1974.

18. Almquist, H.J. "The early history of vitamin K." **American Journal of Clinical Nutrition**, 28, 656-659, 1975.

19. Smith-Barbaro, P., Hanson, D. & Reddy, B.S. "Carcinogen binding to various types of dietary fiber." **Journal of the National Cancer Institute**, 67(2), 495-497, 1981.

20. Wattenberg, L. "Effects of dietary constituents on the metabolism of chemical carcinogens." **Cancer Research**, 35, 3326-3331, 1975.

EYES

HERBS: **EYEBRIGHT** herb (*Euphrasia officinalis*), **Goldenseal root** (*Hydrastis canadensis*), **Bayberry root bark** (*Myrica cerifera*), **Red Raspberry leaves** (*Rubus idaeus*), & **Cayenne** (*Capsicum annum*).

Form: Capsule, Tea

PURPOSE: A tonic for poor or unhealthy vision: (**NOT INTENDED FOR EXTERNAL APPLICATION**); Poor vision.

Other Applications: Preventative treatment for cataracts; blindness, inflamed eyes, stinging and weeping eyes, over-sensitivity to light.

USE: 1. Normal use: 2-4 caps/day.
2. Acute problems: 2-3 caps, three times per day.
3. Use the INFLUENZA or FEVERS & INFECTIONS blends to supplement this blend whenever infection is present.

Contraindications: None. **NOT INTENDED FOR EXTERNAL APPLICATION.**

The principle action of this blend is a tonic to the eyes and the major effect is supplied by Eyebright and Goldenseal. The other herbs in the blend are antibiotics, astringents and stimulants. They provide the "housekeeping" chores for the blend, toning, warding off bacteria, delivering nutrients, and eliminating wastes. Although from time to time one hears reports that blends such as this have cured blindness, cataracts and other severe vision problems, documentation of the diagnostic measures and exact mode of treatment in such cases has been lacking.

EYEBRIGHT, as its name indicates, is one of the primary herbal sources of eye care. Eyebright has been depended upon for at least 2000 years in the treatment of eye problems. Positive clinical cases abound, and glowing personal reports are received by doctors continually. Most cases involve sore and/or inflamed eyes in which there is considerable stinging and irritation associated with watery-to-thick discharges, or conjunctivitis (pink eye). The herb may help to relieve other symptoms that often accompany inflammed eyes, such as runny nose, earache and sneezing. Science has been remiss in not investigating this herb. Eyebright may be procured and used by itself as an eyewash or compress to potentiate the effects of this blend (do not use powdered herb for this purpose; use whole herb). Its mode of action is not known, but used internally, it probably affects the liver among other organs in such a way as to cleanse the blood supply to the eyes.

GOLDENSEAL ROOT, because of its potent antibiotic and antiseptic nature, will greatly help reduce infection and inflammation of the eyes (**1-2**). Herbalists have used Goldenseal in America for over a hundred years for inflammation of the eyes (**3**) and to soothe and tone catarrhal and follicular conjunctivitis (**4**). The American Indians were the first to use it for sore eyes. Early pioneers, along with many Indian tribes, used it as a general tonic, but thought of it as being a specific treatment for the eyes. *(See also INFLUENZA; STOMACH/INTESTINAL; VAGINAL YEAST INFECTION; NERVES & GLANDS; FEVERS & INFECTIONS; HEMORRHOIDS)*

BAYBERRY ROOT BARK is provided in this blend as a stimulating tonic for the good of the whole system. It works well in conjunction with Cayenne to increase the body's ability to ward off infections of all kinds. The tonic and astringent properties of this herb are discussed in the INFLUENZA chapter.

RED RASPBERRY LEAF, in the small quantities found in this blend, imparts a certain amount of astringency to the blend, and is included for that reason. Astringency helps lessen the severity of mucous discharge from, in this case, the eyes and nose. *(See also DIABETES; MENSTRUATION; FEMALE TONIC)*

CAYENNE insures the rapid delivery of nutrients to infected areas as well as the efficient removal of waste material. Such service can be extremely important in cases of eye infection and other eye-related problems. The mode of action of Cayenne is to stimulate the cardio-vascular system as a whole, but is felt predominantly in the capillaries, i.e., precisely where needed for proper infusion of the diseased area with a constant fresh supply of blood-borne nutrients. *(See also CIRCULATION; BLOOD PURIFICATION/DETOXIFICATION; FATIGUE; HIGH BLOOD PRESSURE)*

OTHER NUTRIENTS

VITAMINS
(Daily requirements unless otherwise noted)
Vitamin A *25,000-50,000 I.U.*
Vitamin B Complex
Vitamin B1 *25-50 mg*
Vitamin B2 *25-50 mg*
Vitamin B6 *25-50 mg*
Vitamin C *3,000-5,000 mg*
Vitamin D *400-1,000 I.U.*
Pantothenic Acid *100 mg*
Niacinamide *50 mg*

MINERALS
Calcium/Magnesium
Phosphorous

MISCELLANEOUS
B-Carotene

REFERENCES

1. Gibbs, O.S. "On the curious pharmacology of hydrastis." **Federation of American Societies for Experimental Biology. Federation Proceedings**, 6(1), 332, 1947.
2. Nandkarni, A.K. **Indian Materia Medica**. Popular Book Depot, Bombay-7. Dhootopapeshwar Prakashan Ltd, Panvel 1954, Vol 1. 3rd ed., 189-190.
3. Ellingwood, F. **American Materia Medica, Therapeutics and Pharmacognosy.** Eclectic Medical Publications, Portland, Oregon, 1983.
4. Felter, H. W. **The Eclectic Materia Medica, Pharmacology and Therapeutics.** Eclectic Medical Publications, Portland, Oregon, 1983 (first published 1922).

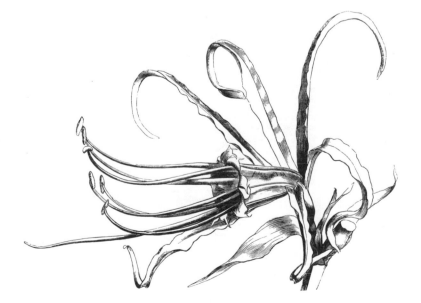

FATIGUE

HERBS: **CAYENNE** (*Capsicum annum*), **Siberian GINSENG** (*Eleutherococcus senticosus*), **Gotu Kola** (*Hydrocotyle asiatica*), **Kelp** (*Laminaria, Macrocystis, Ascophyllum*), **Peppermint leaves** (*Mentha piperita*), **Ginger root** (*Zingiber officinale*).

Form: Capsule.

PURPOSE: Fatigue; Physical weakness; Lack of strength and stamina.

Other Applications: Depression, emotional exhaustion.

USE:
1. Routine Maintenance: 2-4 caps/day.
2. Severe stress: 4-6 caps/day.
3. As adjunct to NERVOUS TENSION blend: 1-2 caps/day.
4. With MENTAL ALERTNESS/SENILITY blend: 2 caps/day.
5. As adjunct to LOW BLOOD SUGAR blend: 1-2 caps/day.

Contraindications: None.

Everybody feels worn out at one time or another, but constant fatigue is a sign of undue physiological stress, whether from overwork or disease. This herbal blend is designed to be a part of a program for overcoming the effects of stress. It promotes both short-term and long-term anti-fatigue properties and enhancement of physical strength and stamina. The Cayenne and Peppermint provide a quick stimulant effect, and when the blend is used daily, the Ginseng, Gotu Kola, Kelp and Ginger root gradually increase stamina.

CAYENNE's stimulant effects have been shown through animal studies to be rapid but transient. Animals, stressed under various conditions, perform better if Cayenne is added to their diet on the day before the tests, but not if added three days before the test (**1**). Animal tests have also demonstrated long-term resistance to stress when Ginseng and Gotu Kola form a semi-permanent part of the diet (**1-2**). In addition, Cayenne has been proven to have a strong effect on circulation and respiratory reflexes (**3**). *(See also CIRCULATION; HIGH BLOOD PRESSURE)*

SIBERIAN GINSENG resembles other Ginseng species in overall activity, though there are some minor differences. Ginseng is properly the number one tonic herb in the world. Used on a daily basis, it gradually builds up the body's ability to resist fatigue. You may find yourself just as tired at the end of the day, but you will have done so much more for it. That is the marvel of Ginseng. Studies on the anti-fatigue (or anti-stress) properties are substantial (e.g.,**4-5**). Ginseng directly stimulates the adrenocortical system (**6**), which helps prevent the cumulative effect of hundreds of different kinds of daily stress from overwhelming the body's ability to fight back. In the aged, Ginseng saponins (the active principles) impart to the body's organs an increased ability to tolerate anaerobic conditions. The result is that ageing heart and brain tissues are better able to withstand sustained work (**7**). *(See also INFERTILITY; WHOLE BODY; MENTAL ALERTNESS/SENILITY; LOW BLOOD SUGAR)*

GOTU KOLA is another tonic of Asian origin. Several years ago I studied Gotu Kola, Ginseng and Capsicum in a blend and separately. I noticed that Gotu Kola behaved similar to Ginseng with regard to effects on fatigue. What little other research has been done agrees with that finding (**8,2**). Contrary to the misconceptions of some writers, including university professors in California and Utah, Gotu Kola is not related to the Kola nut, nor does it owe its anti-fatigue properties to caffeine, a stimulant not found in Gotu Kola. *(See also WHOLE BODY; MENTAL ALERTNESS/SENILITY)*

KELP influences the body first through nutritive excellence, supplying a long list of essential vitamins and mineral salts Secondly, Kelp contains cardiac principles which stimulate the heart ever so gently (**9**).

PEPPERMINT LEAF provides a refreshing aromatic principle to the blend, making the preparation much more acceptable to the body, more digestible, and more utilizable by the body's major systems. In addition, the volatile oils of Peppermint are said to be directly stimulating to the entire body. *(See also DIGESTION; MENTAL ALERTNESS/SENILITY)*

GINGER ROOT produces a generalized stimulant effect on the entire body, and has a few specific properties also. Cardiotonic activity has been noted by Russian and Japanese researchers (**10-11**). Cholinergic properties of the herb help the body recover from the effects of stress and fatigue more rapidly than otherwise. Ginger root also stimulates the vasomotor and respiratory centers (**12**). *(See also NERVOUS TENSION; LOW BLOOD SUGAR; CIRCULATION; LAXATIVE; STOMACH/INTESTINAL; NAUSEA; DIGESTION)*

OTHER NUTRIENTS

VITAMINS
(Daily requirements unless otherwise noted)
Vitamin B-1 *25-100 mg*
Vitamin B-2 *25-100 mg*
Vitamin B-6 *25-100 mg*
Vitamin C *500-1000 mg*
Vitamin D *400 I.U.*
Vitamin E *500-600 I.U.*
Niacinamide *100 mg*
Folic acid *400 mcg*
Pantothenic Acid *100 mg*

MINERALS
Calcium/Magnesium
Phosphorus
Zinc

REFERENCES

1. Mowrey, D.B. "Capsicum, ginseng and gotu kola in combination." **The Herbalist**, premier issue, 22-28, 1975.
2. Mowrey, D.B. "The effects of capsicum, gotu kola and ginseng on activity: further evidence." **The Herbalist**, 1(1), 51-54, 1976.
3. Molnar, E., Baraz, L.A. & Khayutin, V.M. "Irritating and depressing effect of capsaicin on receptors and afferent fibers of the small intestine." **Tr. Inst. Norm. Patol. Fiziol. Akad. Med. Nauk SSSR**, 10, 22-24, 1967.
4. Takagi, K., Saito, H. & Nabata, H. "Pharmacological studies of Panax ginseng root." **Japanese Journal of Pharmacology**, 22, 245-259, 1972.
5. Saito, H., Yoshida, Y. & Takagi, K. "Effect of Panax ginseng on exhaustive exercise in mice." **Japanese Journal of Pharmacology**, 24, 119-127, 1974.
6. Hiai, S. Yokoyama, H., Oura, H. & Yano, S. "Stimulation of pituitary-adrenocortical system by ginseng saponins." **Endocrinologia Japonica**, 26(6), 661-665, 1979.
7. Shia, G.T.W., Ali, S. & Bittles, A.H. "The effects of Ginseng saponins on the growth and metabolism of human diploid fibroblasts." **Gerontology**, 28, 121-124, 1982.
8. List, P.H. & Hoerhammer, L. **Hagers Handbuch der Pharmazeutischen Praxis.** Volumes 2-5, Springer-Verlag, Berlin.
9. Kosuge, T., Nukaya, H., Yamamoto, T. & Tsuji, K. "Isolation and identification of cardiac principles from laminaria." **Yakugaku Zasshi**, 103(6), 683-685, 1983.
10. Khmetova, B.K. "The electrocardiographic changes in patients with chronic pulmonary and pulmonary-cardiac insufficiency treated with European wild ginger." **Sbornik Nauchnykh Trudov Bashkirskii Meditsinskii Institut**, 17, 113-118, 1968.
11. Shoji, N., Iwasa, A., Takemoto, T., Ishida, Y. & Ohizumi, Y. "Cardiotonic principles of ginger (Zingiber officinale, R)." **Journal of Pharmaceutical Science**, 71(10), 1174-1175, 1968.
12. Ally, M.M. "The pharmacological action of zingiber officinale." **Proceedings of the Pan Indian Ocean Scientific Congress, 4th, Karachi, Pakistan**, Section G, 11-12, 1960.

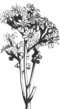

FEMALE TONIC

HERBS: **BLACK COHOSH** root (*Cimicifuga racemosa*), **LICORICE** root (*Glycyrrhiza glabra*), **Raspberry leaves** (*Rubus idaeus*), **Passion Flower** (*Passiflora incarnata*), **Chamomile** (*Matricaria chamomilla*), **Fenugreek** (*Trigonella Foenum-graecum*), **Black Haw bark** (*Viburnum prunifolium*), **Saw Palmetto berries** (*Serenoa repens-sabal*), **Squaw vine** (*Mitchella repens*), **Wild Yam root** (*Dioscorea villosa*), & **Kelp** (*Laminaria, Macrocystis, Ascophyllum*).

Form: Capsule, Tea, Douche

PURPOSE: Female Tonic. For use during pregnancy, delivery, menses, menopause; also for pain, cramp, atony, etc.

Other Applications: Morning Sickness; Hot flashes; Infertility; mild sedative.

USE: 1. As a Tonic: 2-3 caps/day along with 2 caps/day of the NERVE & GLAND TONIC.
2. Menses: 4-6 caps/day.
3. Pregnancy: 3-5 caps/day. Supplement with the NERVE & GLAND TONIC and WHOLE BODY TONIC, 2-3 caps each/day.
4. For morning sickness: use NAUSEA blend as directed; supplement with 3-5 caps/day of this blend.

Contraindications: Persons with low blood sugar should supplement with the LOW BLOOD SUGAR Blend.

The focus of this blend is on sustaining women during pregnancy, parturition, menopause, menstruation, etc. It reduces pain, cramping, atony, etc., and helps maintain good hormonal health and balance. Use the blend moderately on a regular basis. The estrogenic activity of blends such as this one are often exaggerated. Some estrogenic activity may be present, but it is small compared to that derived from estrogen supplments.

BLACK COHOSH promotes and/or restores healthy menstrual activity; it soothes irritation and congestion of the uterus, cervix and vagina; it relieves the pain and distress of pregnancy; it contributes to quick, easy and uncomplicated deliveries; and it promotes uterine involution and recovery (e.g.,**1**). In support of the above clinical evidence, laboratory research has found hypotensive principles, vasodilatory, anti-inflammatory, and uterine contractile activity in Black Cohosh (e.g., **2-3**). *(See also NERVOUS TENSION; HIGH BLOOD PRESSURE)*

LICORICE ROOT's estrogenic activity has been clearly established by experimental investigation (e.g., **4-5**). In a typical animal study, castrated mice and infantile rats are administered various Licorice root extracts, after which the effects of the extracts are measured as, for example, by increased uterine weight. In a study involving women who could not ovulate, normal ovulation was successfully induced, by utilizing an extract of Licorice Root (**6**). *(See also ARTHRITIS; RESPIRATORY AILMENTS; SKIN; BLOOD PURI/DETOX; CIRCULATION; FATIGUE; WEIGHT LOSS; ENVIRONMENTAL POLLUTION; FEVERS & INFECTIONS; THYROID; DETOXIFY/NURTURE; WHOLE BODY; MENTAL ALERTNESS/SENILITY)*

RASPBERRY LEAF is one of those herbs that just seem to be peculiarly well-suited for women. Its effect can best be described as normalization. Raspberry leaf tempers the effects of hormonal runaway, such as might occur during menstruation, pregnancy and delivery. One study showed that Raspberry leaf prevented the typical hypergrowth effects of chronic gonadotrophin on ovaries and uterus (**7**), while another study demonstrated that Raspberry leaf will, in fact, relax uterine muscles (**8**).

PASSION FLOWER can be used to calm nerves that get on edge during the periods of hormonal adjustment common to most women. An analgesic (pain-killing) effect has also been demonstrated in laboratory and clinical tests (**9**). These properties of Passion Flower reduce many of the discomforts of menses, parturition and menopause. *(See also NERVOUS TENSION; INSOMNIA)*

CHAMOMILE possesses a definite and proven uterine tonic property (**10**). Also well-documented are the mild sedative and anti-inflammatory properties of Chamomile (e.g, **11**). One can expect a nice positive interaction between the effects of Passion Flower and Chamomile. Other documented properties of Passion Flower include antispasmotic, carminative, antibacterial, antimycotic, nontoxic, dermatological (**12**). *(See also NERVES & GLANDS)*

FENUGREEK seeds impart tonus to the uterus through a general stimulant action (**13**). While yams are the main source of substances from which sex hormones are made (see below), Fenugreek seeds are currently being cultivated for this purpose (**14**). In Mediterranean countries the seeds are often used to stimulate lactation. As a specific for female problems, Fenugreek thus commands a high position. *(See also CHOLESTEROL REGULATION; STOMACH/INTESTINAL)*

BLACK HAW BARK is an effective treatment for dysmenorrhea, amenorrhea, and threatened abortion (**15**). A definite antispasmodic property has also been established. The herb stabilizes tonus and reduces the severity of contractions (**16**). We would expect this herb to be particularly effective against all forms of menstruation disorders, the anemia of pregnancy, disrupted estrus cycles, and disorders of sexual performance.

SAW PALMETTO BERRY functions as a nutritive tonic, increasing the size and secreting ability of the mammary glands, decreasing ovarian and uterine irritability, relieving dysmenorrhea resulting from lack of tonus, and ameliorating ovarian dysfunction. It is used to treat virtually all diseases of the reproductive system. *(See also INFERTILITY; RESPIRATORY AILMENTS; DIABETES; PROSTATE; NERVES & GLANDS; THYROID; DIGESTION)*

WILD YAM ROOT saponins and derivatives are used to manufacture progesterone, an intermediate in cortisone production. Steroid drugs derived from diosgenin include corticosteroids, oral contraceptives, androgens and estrogens (Yams do not contain, as sometimes believed, full-blown estrogens or other hormones—these substances are produced after four processing steps). Such findings might help explain why, during the previous two centuries of American medicine, Wild Yam roots had successfully been employed in treating dysmenorrhea, ovarian neuralgia and cramps, after pains, and other problems of menses and child-birth. *(See also LIVER DISORDERS)*

KELP is included in this blend, not only for its considerable nutritive and tonic value, but because it performs one other function of great value for women. It prevents breast cancer (**17**). Mild protection for most people can be expected through use of this blend, but if you suspect you need extra protection or insurance, consider taking supplemental Kelp along with this blend. For more information on the anti-cancer properties of Kelp, see ENVIRONMENTAL POLLUTION. *(See also FEVERS & INFECTIONS; WEIGHT LOSS; FATIGUE; BLOOD PURI/DETOX; HEART; INFERTILITY; PAIN; MENTAL ALERTNESS/SENILITY; THYROID; CIRCULATION; DIABETES)*

OTHER NUTRIENTS

VITAMINS

Vitamin A *25,000 I.U.*	Vitamin D *4,000 I.U.*
Vitamin B1 *25-50 mg*	Vitamin E *600-800 I.U.*
Vitamin B2 *25-50 mg*	Folic Acid *400 mcg*
Vitamin B6 *25-50 mg*	Bioflavanoids
Vitamin B12 *up to 50 mcg*	PABA
Vitamin C *1,000 mg*	

MINERALS

Iron
Iodine
Calcium/Magnesium

MISCELLANEOUS

Brewer's yeast	Milk
Kelp	Wheat germ
Cod Liver Oil	

REFERENCES

1. Porcher, F.P "Report on the indigenous medical plants of South Carolina." **Transactions of the American Medical Association.** Vol II, 1849.
2. Young, J. **American Journal of Medical Science.** 9,310, 1831.
3. Farnsworth, N.R. & Seligman, A.B. "Hypoglycemic plants." **Tile and Till,** 57(3), 52-56, 1971.
4. Sharaf, A., Gomaa, N., El-Camal, M.H.A. "Glycyrrhetic acid as an active estrogenic substance separated from glycyrrhiza glabra (liquorice)." **Egyptian Journal of Pharmaceutical Science.** 16 (2), 245-251, 1975.
5. Costello, C.H. & Lynn, E.V. "Estrogenic substances from plants: glycyrrhiza glabra." **Journal of the American Pharmaceutical Association.** 39, 177-180, 1950.
6. Yaginuma, T; Izumi, R., Yasui, H., Arai, T. & Kawabata, M. "Effect of traditional herbal medicine on serum testosterone levels and its induction of regular ovulation in hyper-androgenic and oligomenorrhetic women." **Nippon Sanka Fujinka Gakkai Zasshi,** 34(7), 939-944, 1982.
7. Kurzepa, S. & Samojlik, E. "The effect of extracts from some Rosaceae plants upon the gonadotrophic and thyrotrophic activities in rat." **Endokrynologia Polska.** 15(2), 143-150, 1963.
8. Burn, J.H. & Withell, E.R. "A principle in rasberry leaves which relaxes uterine muscles." **Lancet.** 2(6149), 1-3, 1941.
9. Ambuhl, H. "Anatomische und chemische untersuchungen an Passiflora coerulea L., und Passiflor incarnata L." Dissertation Number 3830 ETH, Zurich, 1966.
10. Shipochliev, T. "Extracts from a group of medicinal plants enhancing uterine tonus." **Veterinary Sciences (Sofia).** 18(4), 94-98, 1981.
11. Breinlich, J. & Scharnagel, K. "Pharmacological properties of the ene-yne dicycloethers from matricaria chamomilla. antiinflammatory , antianaphylactic, spasmolytic, and bacteriostatic activity." **Arzneimittel-Forschungen,** 18(4), 429-431, 1968.
12. Demling, L. **Erfahrungstherapie—spaete Rechtfertigung.** Verlag G. Braun, Karlsruhe, West Germany, 1975.
13. Arbo & Al-Kafawi. **Plant Medica.** 17, 14, 1969.
14. Thomson, W.A.R. **Herbs that Heal.** Charles Scribner's Sons, New York, 1976, pp. 160-161.
15. List, P.H. & Hoerhammer, L. **Hagers Handbuch der Pharmazeutischen Praxis.** Volumes 2-5, Springer-Verlag, Berlin.
16. Horhammer, L., Wagner, H. & Reinhardt, H. "Chemistry, pharmacology, and pharmaceutics of the components from viburnam prunifolium and v. opulus." **Botanical Magazine (Tokyo),** 79, 510-525, 1966.
17. Teas, J. "The dietary intake of *Laminaria*, a brown seaweed, and breast cancer prevention." **Nutrition and Caner.** 4(3), 217-223, 1983.

FEVERS & INFECTIONS

HERBS: **ECHINACEA root** (*Echinacea Purpurea*), **MYRRH gum** (*Commiphora myrrha*), **Goldenseal root** (*Hydrastis canadensis*), **Licorice root** (*Glycyrrhiza glabra*), **Blue Vervain** (*Verbena hastata*), **Cinchona** (*Peruvian bark*), **Butternut root bark** (*Juglans cinerea*), **Garlic** (*Allium sativum*) & **Kelp** (*Laminaria, Macrocystis, Ascophyllum*).

Form: Capsule, Tea, Compress, Poultice

PURPOSE: To alleviate fevers (general ailments due to common colds and influenza); Infections.

Other Applications: Parasites, amoebic infections.

USE: 1. Fevers: 3 caps, 4 times/day with plenty of liquid.

2. Infections: *Internal*—anywhere from 2 - 12 caps/day. *External*—2-3 caps applied as a poultice or wash. Consider adding Chaparral to this poultice.

3. Use NAUSEA blend if necessary.

4. For cleanses, use 2-3 capsules per day in conjunction with the DETOXIFY/NURTURE blend, as directed.

Contraindications: None.

This blend kills germs that cause fevers and infections. It increases the body's resistance, increases the body's capacity to withstand a successful invasion, and boosts the body's ability to recuperate. Fevers of all kinds, including the rare typhoid, malaria, and meningitis, have been successfully treated and/or prevented by these herbs.

ECHINACEA destroys the germs of infection directly, and bolsters the body's defenses by magnifying the white blood cell count (**1**). In recent years, research has discovered the mechanisms by which Echinacea may work to prevent infection (**2**). The herb acts to effectively close down one of the major routes of bug-invasion, and it inhibits the spread of infection that may have already occurred. Cortisone-like activity has also been discovered in Echinacea (**3**), and the herb accelerates the production of granulomatous tissue (necessary for healing) and has a stimulating effect on the lymph system (**4**). *(See also SKIN DISORDERS; BLOOD PURIFICATION/DETOXIFICATION)*

MYRRH GUM contains many familiar volatile oils which make the herb ideally suited for promoting free breathing during congestive colds, and for clearing out mucous-clogged passages throughout the body (**5**). It increases circulation by stimulating capillary activity, restores tone and normal secretion, increase digestion, promotes the absorption and assimilation of nutrients, increases the number of white blood cells, and through all of these means is helpful in treating feverish symptoms like cold skin, weak pulse, and so on (**1,4,6**). *(See also STOMACH/INTESTINAL)*

GOLDENSEAL ROOT is a proven antibiotic and antiseptic. See the INFLUENZA chapter for a further discussion.

LICORICE ROOT has the ability to prevent and remedy infections, inflammations and fevers. It has antibacterial activity against several common gram negative intestinal pathogens (**7**), and antiviral activity of considerable potency (**8-9**). Licorice root constituents actually activate the interferon mechanism (**12**). Several studies have been published that underscore the anti-inflammatory property of Licorice root (e.g., **10-11**), an effect that is directly related to the herb's corticosteroid-like action. It is an important characteristic for it helps the body deal with the inflammation that often accompanies various infections. *(See also ARTHRITIS; RESPIRATORY AILMENTS; SKIN DISORDERS; FEMALE TONIC; DETOXIFY/NURTURE)*

BLUE VERVAIN is added to many blends to impart its own special stimulant properties. During convalescence, one should be sure to include this herb in the diet. The herb possesses noticeable anti-inflammatory and analgesic properties (**13**) which are extremely useful in curbing infectious swelling and pain. Blue Vervain is recommended as a diaphoretic (to make a feverish person sweat) and as an expectorant to relieve cold symptoms. *(See also NERVES & GLANDS)*

CINCHONA, the primary source for quinine until the drug was synthetically produced, possesses the same antiviral, antimalarial, antipyretic properties as the drug. An effective dose of Cinchona extract elicits the same antimalarial activity as an effective dose of quinine (**14**). Though large doses of Cinchona have a depressant effect on the heart, small amounts are completely harmless. Before the advent of quinine-the drug, Americans used Cinchona not only for malaria and other fevers, but also as a tonic, and to stimulate the appetite and digestion (**15**).

BUTTERNUT ROOT BARK is used in this blend primarily for its mild laxative property. Its inclusion conforms to the principle of balance in herbal blending which states that in blends dealing with combat of infections, fevers and colds, some part of the treatment should be laxative to help the body rid itself of bacteria-laden wastes. *(See also LAXATIVE; PARASITES)*

GARLIC is sometimes reported to be more effective than penicillin for the treatment of fevers, throat infections, and other infectious disease (**16**). It is a noteworthy antibiotic against bacilli and germs that cause any number of ailments. The antibacterial, antiviral and antifungal activity of Garlic have been proven against numerous organisms including *Candida Albicans*, the organism that causes most cases of vaginitis (vaginal yeast infection). Athlete's foot fungus and at least 20 other pathogenic fungi are susceptible to destruction by the antimicrobial property of Garlic. In a most remarkable study, the herb was found 100% effective against the usually fatal cryptococcal meningitis (**17**). Garlic is also able to protect living organisms against influenza virus (**18**). The above review is but a sample of the available research along these lines. *(See also HIGH BLOOD PRESSURE; PARASITES)*

KELP also helps ward off infections and fevers. It works by killing various gram positive and gram negative bacteria, including many of those already enumerated (**19**). In addition to these direct effects, Kelp is, of course, very helpful in terms of supplying nutritional support for the ailing and convalescent patient. *(See also FATIGUE; BLOOD PURIFICATION/DETOXIFICATION)*

OTHER NUTRIENTS

VITAMINS
(Daily requirements unless otherwise noted)

Vitamin A 25,000-50,000 I.U.	Vitamin C 3,000-5,000 mg
Vitamin B Complex	500 mg/hour—1st day
Vitamin B1 25-100 mg	Vitamin D 400-600 I.U.
Vitamin B2 25-100 mg	Pantothenic Acid 50 mg
Vitamin B6 25-100 mg	Niacinamide 50 mg

MINERALS
Calcium/Magnesium
Phosphorus
Potassium
Sodium

MISCELLANEOUS
Cod Liver Oil
GLA
Essential Fatty Acid
HCl

REFERENCES

1. Ellingwood, F. **American Materia Medica, Therapeutics and Pharmacognosy.** Eclectic Medical Publications, Portland, Oregon, 1983.
2. Bonadeo, I., Bottazzi, G. & Lavazza, M. "Echinacina B: polisaccaride attiva dell' Echinacea." **Rev. Ital. Essenze Profumi**, 53, 281, 1971.
3. Keller, H. "Recovery of active agents from aqueous extracts of the species of echinacea." **Ger. 950,674**, Oct 11, 1956.
4. List, P.H. & Hoerhammer, L. **Hagers Handbuch der Pharmazeutischen Praxis.** Volumes 2-5, Springer-Verlag, Berlin.
5. Leung, A.Y. **Encyclopedia of Common Natural Ingredients.** New York, 1980.
6. Tyler, V.E., Brady, L.R. & Robbers, J.E. **Pharmacognosy**, 7th Edition, Lea & Febiger, Philadelphia, 1976.
7. Kou-sheng, L. & Chang, P.W.H. "In vitro antibacterial activity of some common chinese herbs on gram negative intestinal pathogens." **Chinese Medical Journal**, 68, 307-312, 1950.
8. Pompei, R., Pnie, A., Flore, O., Marcialis, M.A., & Loddo, B. "Antiviral activity of glycyrrhizic acid." **Experientia**, 36, 304, 1980.
9. Pompei, R., Flore, O., Marccialis, M.A., Pani, A., & Loddo, B. "Glycyrrhetinic acid inhibits virus growth and inactivates virus particles." **Nature**, 281, 689-690, 1979.
10. Finney, S.H. & Somers, G.F. "The anti-inflammatory activity of glycyrrhetinic acid and derivatives." **Journal of Pharmacology and Pharmacodynamics**, 10(10), 613-620, 1958.
11. Tangri, K.K., Seth, P.K., Parmar, S.S. & Bhargava, K.P. "Biochemical study of anti-inflammatory and anti-arthritic properties of glycyrrhetic acid." **Biochemical Pharmacology**, 14(8), 1277-1281, 1965.
12. Abe, N. Ebina, T. & Ishida, N. "Interferon induction by glycyrrhizin and glycyrrhetinic acid in mice." **Microbiology and Immunology**, 26(6), 535-539, 1982.
13. Sakai, S. "Pharmacological actions of verbena officinalis." **Gifu Ika Daigaku Kiyo**, 11(1), 6-17, 1963.
14. Aviado, D.M., Rosen, T., Dacanay, H. & Plotkin, S.H. "Antimalarial and antiarrhythmic activity of plant extracts." **Medicina Experimentalis—International Journal of Experimental Medicine**, 19(2), 79-94, 1969.
15. Osol, A., Pratt, R. & Altschule, M.D. **The United States Dispensatory and Physicians' Pharmacology**, 26 ed., J.B. Lippincott Co., Phila.
16. Fortunatov, M.N. "Experimental use of phytoncides for therapeutic and prophylactic purpose." **Voprosy Pediatrii i Okhrany Materinstva: Detstva**, 20(2), 55-58, 1952.
17. Hunan Medical College, China. "Garlic in cryptococcal meningitis. A preliminary report of 21 cases." **Chinese Medical Journal**, 93, 123-126, 1980.
18. Nagai, K. "Experimental studies on the preventive effect of garlic extract against infection with influenza virus." **Japanese Journal of the Association for Infectious Diseases**, 47, 111-115, 1973.
19. Mautner, H.G., Gardner, G.M. & Pratt, R. "Antibiotic activity of seaweed extracts." **Journal of the American Pharmaceutical Association**, 42(5), 294-296, 1953.

HAYFEVER AND ALLERGIES

HERBS: **CLAY** (*Montmorillonite*), **Wild Cherry bark** (*Prunus serotina*), **Mullein leaves** (*Verbascum thapsus*), & **Horehound** (*Marrubium vulgare*).

Form: Capsule, Gargle

PURPOSE: To prevent the symptoms of allergies: use if you are susceptible to hayfever, asthma, food allergies, chemical allergies, etc.

Other Applications: None.

USE: 1. Hayfever: 1 cap several times per day, starting two weeks before hayfever season. Reduce use to 1 cap two to three times per day during the season.

2. Food Allergies: 3-4 caps at first sign (or sooner if possible), and 1 cap every 1-2 hours during reaction period.

3. Misc. Allergies (dust, animal, etc.): 1-2 caps every 1-2 hours during exposure to allergen. **NOTE:** Drink 1/2 cup liquid whenever ingesting these capsules.

Contraindications:

This blend can best be described as preventive. The idea is to stop allergic reactions to inhalant and ingestive allergens before they happen. Once the antigen-antibody reaction takes place, there is little that can be done to prevent an allergic reaction. This blend is designed to prevent that reaction from taking place. Remember it will be most effective if used *prior to* as well as *during* hayfever season.

MONTMORILLONITE CLAY is highly **ad**sorbent (not **ab**sorbent). By quickly neutralizing allergens before these foreign invaders can attach themselves to blood cells, adsorptive surfaces prevent allergic reactions. That is the purpose of the clay. Water soluble allergens are also bound up by the clay due to its intense hydrophyllic (water-loving) nature. Therefore, to ingest bentonite in a pre-hydrated gel form would be a mistake if you are trying to prevent allergies, since the gel would not be able to adsorb many more allergen-bearing water molecules. The substantiation of these facts comes from several different sources (e.g., **1-3**). The quality, or ionic makeup, of the clay is very important (**4**), the better clays being predominantly sodium montmorillonite.

WILD CHERRY BARK is an excellent calming and soothing agent for irritated mucosal surfaces, but would be of little value during an actual allergic reaction. In this blend its primary action is to soothe any mildly irritated surfaces that result from allergens escaping the adsorptive action of the clay. *(See also RESPIRATORY AILMENTS)*

MULLEIN LEAF provides an ounce of mucilaginous protection to mucous surfaces, thereby inhibiting the absorption of allergens through those membranes. During a particular strong exposure to a potent allergen, this bit of protection may make the difference between all allergenic particles being adsorbed or a few making it through and creating distress. *(See also RESPIRATORY AILMENTS; HEMORRHOIDS)*

HOREHOUND affects the respiration directly by dilating vessels (**5**) and acting as a serotonin antagonist (**6**). It should help alleviate any respiratory distress that occurs. Be sure to also use the blend for RESPIRATORY AILMENTS should distress continue or get worse.

OTHER NUTRIENTS

VITAMINS
(Daily requirement unless otherwise noted)
Vitamin A *25,000-50,000 I.U.*
Vitamin B Complex
Vitamin B1 *25-50 mg*
Vitamin B2 *25-50 mg*
Vitamin B6 *25-100 mg*
Vitamin B12 *10 mcg*
Vitamin C *1,000-1,500 mg*
Vitamin D *600 I.U.*
Vitamin E *400-800 I.U.*
Pantothenic acid *150-200 mg*
Choline *1,000 mg*
Inositol *1,000 mg*
Niacinamide *50 mg*

MINERALS
Calcium/Magnesium
Phosphorous
Manganese
Potassium
Sodium

MISCELLANEOUS
Bee Pollen
Liver
HCl

REFERENCES

1. Erschoff, B.H. & Bajwa, G.S. "Physiological effects of dietary clay supplements." Final report on contract number NAS 9-3905, 1965, available from NASA Manned Spacecraft Center, Houston, TX.
2. Smith, R.R. "Recent Advances in nutrition: clay in trout diets." Presented at the USTAFA Convention, no date.
3. Britton, R.A., Dolling, D.P. & Klopfenstein, T.J. "Effect of complexing sodium bentonite with soybean meal or urea in vitro ruminal ammonia release and nitrogen retention in ruminants." **Journal of Animal Science**, 46, 1738, 1978.
4. Lacy, W.J. "Decontamination of radioactively contaminated water by slurrying with clay." **Industrial and Engineering Chemistry**, 45(5), 1061-1065, 1954.
5. Karryev, M.O., Bairyev, C.B., & Ataeva, A.S. "Some therapeutic properties and phytochemistry of common horehound." **Izvestiya Akademiya Nauk Turkmenskoi SSR, Seriya Biologicheskikh Nauk**, 3, 86-88, 1976.
6. Cahen, R. "Pharmacologic spectrum of marrubium vulgare." **Comptes Rendus des Seances de la Societe de Biolgie et de ses Filiales (Paris)** 164(7), 1467-1472, 1970.

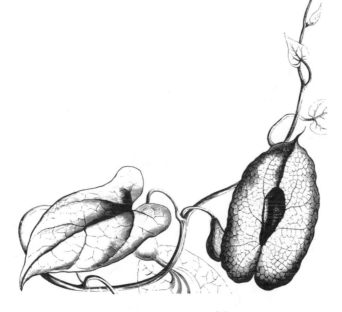

HEART

HERBS: **HAWTHORN** berries (*Crataegus oxyacantha*), **MOTHERWORT** (*Leonurus cardiaca*), **Rosemary leaves** (*Rosmarinus officinalis*), **Kelp** (*Laminara, Macrocystis, Ascophyllum*) & **Cayenne** (*Capsicum annum*).

Form: Capsule.

PURPOSE: Nutritional tonic for the heart.

Other Applications: The use of this blend may help prevent and/or reduce the severity of and/or reduce the symptoms of many heart disease-related conditions. **Consult your physician for any of these conditions. Use this blend as a tonic in long term health programs; do not expect it to "cure" acute episodes**

USE: As Heart tonic: 2-4 caps/day.

Contraindications: None. This is an extremely safe preparation. But it may potentiate the action of digitalis. If you are under the care of a physician, keep him informed about your program so that doses of standard medications may be adjusted as necessary.

This is an interesting blend of herbs designed as a genuine tonic for the heart, not just as a momentary stimulant. The "heart" of this blend is the Hawthorn berry. Motherwort and Rosemary have also been experimentally shown to possess mild cardiotonic and sedative activity, but are more effective when combined with other plants with similar pharmacological activity. Cayenne promotes general increased circulation and catalyzes the chemical reactions of the other herbs. The combining of powdered Cayenne and Hawthorn in a single capsule produces a special kind of synergism that augments the cardiotonic activity of both.

HAWTHORN BERRY functions by 1) peripheral vasodilation, i.e., by dilating the blood vessels away from the heart, thereby lowering the blood pressure and reducing the burden placed on the heart; 2) very mild dilation of coronary vessels; 3) increased enzyme metabolism in the heart muscle, leading to better coronary health; and 4) increased oxygen utilization by the heart (**1-4**). In patients with coronary perfusion disorders one study found a 77% reduction in oxygen utilization with the herb, compared to a 25% reduction with standard forms of treatment (**1**). The study thereby confirmed the oxygen-saving effect of Hawthorn extract on the heart muscle under stress. In almost all patients with primary heart disease, Hawthorn extract produces an improvement in heart dynamics In patients with secondary heart disease the effect is not as great in terms of the number of cases helped, but significant effects are seen in those cases that were helped. The herb has also helped patients whose heart disease is caused by hepatitis or other liver disease. Hawthorn possesses marked vasodilatory action, and lowers peripheral resistance to blood flow (**4**).

Hawthorn appears to have a less immediate effect than digitalis. Unlike digitalis, Hawthorn exhibits an absence of cumulative activity. There is an apparent synergism between Hawthorn Berry and digitalis, as suggested by the fact that heart tissue pretreated with either one becomes sensitized to the other, so that only about half the normal dose of the second is required to obtain normal results (**5**).

MOTHERWORT is one of those plants that has somehow found its way into native medical lore in every corner of the earth from Russia to Rumania, from America to Asia. As a cardiac tonic, Motherwort has been shown to be hypotensive (**6**), sedative (**7**) and antispasmodic. It calms palpitations and normalizes heart function in general. Motherwort extract has been shown to improve several aspects of coronary health (**8**).

ROSEMARY LEAF derivatives possess considerable smooth muscle stimulant activity (and some analgesic activity) (**9**). The herb calms and soothes irritated nerves and upset stomach, and extinguishes strenuous anxiety. (*See also PAIN*)

KELP has proven nutritive (**10**), antibiotic (**11**) and hypotensive (**12**) properties, all of which enhance the cardiotonic effectiveness of the blend. (*See also CIRCULATION; FEVERS & INFECTIONS; WEIGHT LOSS; FATIGUE; BLOOD PURIFICATION/DETOXIFICATION; PAIN; INFERTILITY; MENTAL ALERTNESS/SENILITY; ENVIRONMENTAL POLLUTION; THYROID; DIABETES*)

CAYENNE is the primary stimulant in the blend. Its presence assures the delivery of the other active principles to the vital systems of the body. In addition, it does contain important nutrients for the health of the circulatory system (**13**), such as alpha-tocopherols, vitamin C, minerals and other nutrients.

OTHER NUTRIENTS

VITAMINS
(Daily requirements unless otherwise noted)
  Vitamin A *25,000 I.U. minimum*
  Vitamin B Complex
  Vitamin B12 *25 mcg*
  Vitamin B1 *25-100 mg*
  Vitamin B2 *25-100 mg*
  Vitamin B6 *25-100 mg*
  Vitamin C *1,00-3,000 mg*
  Vitamin D Vitamin E *200-600 I.U.*
  Bioflavanoids *300-600 mg*
  Niacinamide *100 mg*
  Choline *1,000 mg*
  Inositol *1,000 mg*
  PABA
  Pantothenic acid

MINERALS
  Iodine
  Potassium
  Calcium/Magnesium
  Chromium
  Zinc
  Phosphorous

MISCELLANEOUS
  Essential Fatty Acids
  GLA
  Lecithin
  Brewer's Yeast

REFERENCES

1. Kandziora, J. "Crataegutt-wirkung bei koronaren durchblutungsstoerungen." **Muenchener Medizinischer Wochenschrift.** 6, 295-298, 1969.
2. Echte, W. "Die Einwirkung von Weissdorn-extrakten auf die dynamik des menschlichen herzens." (The effect of Hawthorn extracts on the dynamics of the human heart). **Aerztliche Forshung** 14(11), I/560-566, 1960.
3. Ullsperger, R. "Vorlaufige mitteilung ueber den coronargefaesse erweiternden wirkkoerper aus weissdorn." (Preliminary communication concerning a coronary vessel dilating principle from hawthorn). **Pharmazie.** 6(4), 141-144, 1951.
4. Hammerl, H., Kranzl, C., Pichler, O. & Studlar, M. "Klinisch experimentelle stoffwechseluntersuchungen mit einem crataegus extrakt." (Clinical and experimental investigations on metabolism with an extract of Crataegus). **Aerztliche Forshung,** 21(7), 261-270, 1967.
5. Bersin, T., Mueller, A. & Schwarz, H. "Substances contained in crataegus oxyacantha. III. A heptahydroxyflavan glycoside." **Arzneimittel-Forschungen,** 5, 490-491, 1955.
6. Arustamova, F.A. "Hypotensive effect of leonurus cardiaca on animals in experimental chronic hypertension." **Izvestiya Akademii Nauk Armyanski SSR, Biologicheski Nauki.** 16(7), 47-52, 1963.
7. Kubota, S., & Nakashima, S. "The study of leonurus sibericus L. II. Pharmacological study of the alkaloid 'leonurin' isolated from leonurus sibericus L." **Folia Pharmacologica Japonica** 11(2), 159-167, 1930.
8. Xia, Y. X. "The inhibitory effect of Motherwort extract on pulsating myocardial cells in vitro." **Journal of Traditional Chinese Medicine.** 3(3), 185-188, 1983.
9. Boido, A, Sparatore, F, Biniecka, M. "N-substituted derivatives of rosmaricine." **Studi Sassaresi, Sezione 2** (Italian), 53(5-6), 383-393, 1975.
10. Binding, G.J. & Moyle, A. **About Kelp.** Thorsons Publishers Ltd. Wellingborough, England, 1974.
11. Biard, J.F., Verbist, J.F., Boterff, J., Rages, G. & Lecocq, M.M. "Seaweeds of French Atlantic coast with antibacterial and antifungal compounds." **Plant Medica.** Supplement , 136-151, 1980.
12. Funayama, S., & Hikino, H. "Hypotensive principle of laminaria and allied seaweeds." **Planta Medica.** 41, 29-33, 1981.
13. Searl, P.B., Norton, T.R. * Lum, B.K.B. "Study of a cardiotonic fraction from an extract of the seaweed, *Undaria pinnatifida*. **Proceedings of the Western Pharmacology Society.** 24, 63-65, 1981.

HEMORRHOIDS/ASTRINGENT

HERBS: SLIPPERY ELM (*Ulmus vulva*), WITCH HAZEL (*Hamamelis virginiana*), **Mullein** (*Verbascum thapsus*), **Wild Alum** (*Geranium maculatum*), **Goldenseal root** (*Hydrastis canadensis*).

Form: Capsule, Topical, Stiz Bath

PURPOSE: To soothe and heal hemorrhoids; and an effective general astringent for other purposes.

Other Applications: Varicose veins; phlebitis.

USE: 1. Hemorrhoids, internal: 2-4 caps/day.
2. Hemorrhoids, external: Mix with vasoline and apply directly to affected area.
3. Astringent, internal: 1-2 caps as desired.
4. Astringent, external: Make strong tea or poultice and apply to desired area, except eyes.

Contraindications: None.

Hemorrhoids are enlarged veins in the mucous membrane in the rectal area caused by straining against hard, dry stools, by pressure on the veins from an enlarged uterus, by liver disorders, by heart disorders, or by tumors. Relief from the concomitant itching, bleeding, pain and general discomfort is obtained by compresses, sitz baths, analgesic ointments, and by ingesting capsules of herbs that attempt to tone up and remedy the situation from the inside out, by soothing inflamed and sore tissues, shrinking the swollen veins and toning up the body to remove the various causes of hemorrhoids. Each herb in this blend has a history of imparting hemorrhoidal relief. Some of the above herbs have found their way into modern ointments and medications, and this blend can certainly be used in any of the afore-mentioned sitz baths and compresses.

SLIPPERY ELM BARK is used both in poultices and internally to soothe irritated mucous membranes. One early American ethnobotanist described the various uses for Slippery Elm that he observed among the Indians and among the pioneers and settlers of the West as follows: urinary and bowel complaints, sore throat, scurvy, diarrhea, dysentery, cholera infantum, nutritious food, externally for ulcers, tumors, swellings, chillblains, burns and sores (**1**). In all of these uses, the demulcent property of the herb was the therapeutic agent. Slippery Elm was not highly recommended during the last century for hemorrhoids, for it was felt that this particular ailment should be treated primarily with astringents. One exception, a 19th century eclectic physician recommended an external application of Slippery Elm for hemorrhoids (**2**), but this is a rare reference. Modern works are more willing to include the treatment of hemorrhoids as within the realm of demulcents. Certainly, the mucilaginous property of the plant makes it an ideal application for hemorrhoids, both internally and externally. *(See also RESPIRATORY AILMENTS; BONE-FLESH-CARTILAGE)*

WITCH HAZEL LEAF use began with the Indians, and was subsequently adopted by the white community. Now it is the premier treatment for hemorrhoids (**3-4**), finding its place in many currently available hemorrhoid preparations. Its effectiveness is due mainly to its very astringent nature, which, in turn has been attributed to its high content of tannic acid. However, a tannin free Witch Hazel water is also very astringent, so there must be other active principles in the plant. As usual, the whole is better than any of the parts. What laboratory tests have been done, show that Witch Hazel lowers blood pressure, decreases renal volume, accelerates respiration and inhibits peristalsis, indicating a primary effect on the venal system (**5**). This action would help explain why it works so well on hemorrhoids and other venous sicknesses like varicose veins and phlebitis (**6**). Witch Hazel leaf is also bacteriostatic to those surfaces that are washed by it, as has been demonstrated in controlled laboratory studies (**6a-7**). *(See also VAGINAL YEAST INFECTION)*

MULLEIN LEAF, a demulcent, is used externally in poultices and internally in capsules to soothe irritated mucous membranes. The leaf yields a peculiar fatty matter that reduces swelling and pain. In India, Mullein has enjoyed good popularity not only as a demulcent, but also as a bacteriostatic. In that country, and a few others, Mullein has been used to treat tuberculosis for centuries. That practice has found substantiation in laboratory tests wherein Mullein significantly inhibited *mycobacterium tuberculosis* (**8**). *(See also RESPIRATORY AILMENTS; ALLERGY)*

ALUM ROOT, or Cranesbill root, a strong astringent, was introduced to medicine by the American Indians. Knowledgeable American physicians still use it to reduce inflammation of mucous membranes, curb irritation of hemorrhoidal tissue and to restore venous health. It is especially powerful astringent for passive bleeding, as occurs in hematuria, hemoptysis and menorrhagia, and has a potent healing effect on the entire gastrointestinal tract. An early ethnobotanist wrote, "This root is accounted a great medicine by the Meskwaki....Its greatest use is in curing piles and hemorrhoids. A poultice of the pounded root is bound upon the anus to cause protruding piles to recede." (**9**). Like Mullein, it was found to be active against tuberculosis bacteria (**8**). *(See also MENSTRUATION)*

GOLDENSEAL ROOT is, of course, used for many different complaints, hemorrhoids being just one of them. However, it is unclear just how Goldenseal alleviates this condition. One clue is provided by studies that found Goldenseal to constrict peripheral blood vessels (**5, 10-11**). A review of the other sections on Goldenseal in this book will reveal that the herb has profound effects on all parts of the gastrointestinal tract, as well as related systems. Whatever the mechanism, the herb has been successfully used for a couple of hundred years in the United States to reduce the inflammation and pain of hemorrhoidal tissue. *(See also STOMACH/INTESTINAL; INFLUENZA; EYES; VAGINAL YEAST INFECTION; FEVERS & INFECTIONS)*

OTHER NUTRIENTS

VITAMINS
(Daily requirements unless otherwise noted)
Vitamin A *25,000 I.U.*
Vitamin B Complex
Vitamin B1 *25-100 mg*
Vitamin B2 *25-100 mg*
Vitamin B6 *25-100 mg*
Vitamin C *1,000-3,000 mg*
Vitamin D *400 I.U.*
Vitamin E *600 I.U.*
Bioflavonoids

MINERALS
Calcium/Magnesium
Zinc

MISCELLANEOUS
Fluids

REFERENCES

1. Rafinesque, C.S. **Medical fora or manual of medical botany of the United States**, Vol I., 1828, p. 15.
2. Felter, H. W. **The Eclectic Materia Medica, Pharmacology and Therapeutics.** Eclectic Medical Publications, Portland, Oregon, 1983 (first published 1922).
3. Trease, G.E. & Evans, W.C. **Pharmacognosy**, 11th Ed., Bailliere Tindall, London, 1978.
4. **The Dispensatory of the United States of America**, 23rd Ed., Lippincott, Philadelphia, 1943.
5. List, P.H. & Hoerhammer, L. **Hagers Handbuch der Pharmazeutischen Praxis.** Volumes 2-5, Springer-Verlag, Berlin.
6. Mockle, J.A. **Contributions a l'etude des plante medicinales du Canada.** Paris ed. Jouve, p. 63.
6a. D'Amico, M.L. "Ricerche sulla presenza di sostanze ad azione antibiotica nelle piante superiori." **Fitoterapia**, 21(1), 77-79, 1950.
7. Schaufelberger, D. & Hostettmann, K. "On the molluscicidal activity of tannin containing plants." **Planta Medica**, 48, 105-107, 1983.
8. Fitzpatrick, F.K. "Plant substances active against mycobacterium tuberculosis." **Antibiotics and Chemotherapy**, 4(5), 528-536, 1954.
9. Smith, H. **Ethnobotany of the Meskwaki.** Bulletin of Public Museum of Milwaukee 4, 189-274, 1928.
10. Genest, K. & Hughes, D.W. "Natural products in canadian pharmaceuticals." **Canadian Journal of Pharmaceutical Sciences**, 4(2), 41-45, 1969.
11. Ikram, M. "A review of the chemical and pharmacological aspects of genus berberis." **Planta Medica**, 28, 353-358, 1975.

INFERTILITY

HERBS: **DAMIANA** leaves (*Turnera aphrodisiaca*), **GINSENG** (*Siberian*) (*Eleutherococcus senticosus*), **Sarsaparilla root** (*Smilax officinalis*), **Saw Palmetto berries** (*Serenoa serrulata*), **Licorice root** (*Glycyrrhiza glabra*), & **Kelp** (*Laminara, Macrocystis, Asocphyllum*).

Form: Capsule, Tea

PURPOSE: To help assist fertility; To help ameliorate many forms of impotence and related problems.

Other Applications: Hot flashes, vaginal-uterine infections, general tonic, arthritis, rheumatism, menstrual problems.

USE: 1. Infertility: 3-6 caps/day. For best results use every day.
2. In conjunction with the WHOLE BODY TONIC blend, use 2 caps of each per day.
3. For Hot Flashes: Take one caps several times daily during critical periods. Supplement with 3-6 caps/day of the FEMALE TONIC Blend.

Contraindications: None.

While the search for the elusive perfect instantaneous aphrodisiac goes on, it is my contention that the solution to good sexual health lies in possessing and maintaining a sound reproductive system. Of the thousands of plants purported to have aphrodisiac properties, this blend contains only herbs with proven long-term effectiveness in regenerating good hormonal health. Because it enriches the entire genito-urinary and reproductive system, when used regularly, it diminishes the symptoms of arthritis, rheumatism, and especially menstrual problems. Evidence of the blend's effectiveness is provided by basic animal research, human research, clinical trials, cross-cultural verification, and pharmacological investigation.

DAMIANA LEAF has one the strongest reputations for building enhanced sexual activity. This reputation extends over hundreds of years. Damiana's use as an aphrodisiac can be traced to the ancient Mayans (**1**), but in Modern times it is also popularly used as a sexual stimulant (**2**). Damiana leaf contains beta-sitosterol and various aromatic oils that could have some stimulant effect on the sexual apparatus or could help build sexual health and reproductivity.

SIBERIAN GINSENG's centuries-old aphrodisiac use is known to almost everybody—indeed, highly controlled research from Japan and Korea has substantially verified that effect (e.g., **3**). The general tonic and anti-stress properties of Ginseng contribute to the overall health required of the body for proper sexual functioning (**4**). (*See also FATIGUE, WHOLE BODY, MENTAL ALERTNESS/SENILITY, BLOOD SUGAR*)

SAW PALMETTO BERRY is often used in conjunction with Damiana to promote sexual health. Historically, Saw Palmetto berries were used in America to treat several related disorders of the genito-urinary system, including inflammation, rupture and blockage (**5**). At least one authority from those years testified to its salving effect on gonorrhea (**6**). (*See also RESPIRATORY AILMENTS, DIABETES, FEMALE TONIC, PROSTATE, NERVES & GLANDS, THYROID, DIGESTION*)

SARSAPARILLA ROOT is used in the treatment of venereal disease and infertility in Honduras, Mexico, the United States, South America and China, and elsewhere, and by the North American Indians (**7**). The steroid saponins and genins of Sarsaparilla closely resemble, and are used in the synthesis of, steroid sex hormones. Preparations containing Sarsaparilla as the primary agent are commonly used in China in the treatment of syphilis with reported success rates as high as 90% (**8**). (*See also ARTHRITIS, BLOOD PURIFICATION/DETOXIFICATION, WHOLE BODY, DETOXIFY/NURTURE*)

LICORICE ROOT contains an estrogenic activity that was first discovered in 1950 (**9**). In 1963, a report appeared revealing a very strong estrogenic activity in Egyptian Licorice Root (**10**). Two tests, one in 1975 (**11**) and one in 1979 (**12**), found contradictory evidence concerning the estrogenic properties of glycyrrhizin (a crude extract of Licorice Root). Those studies suggest that more work, utilizing *whole* herb should be done. In a very recent study on women experiencing infrequent menstruation, a Licorice Root preparation successfully induced normal ovulation (**13**). (*See also*

ARTHRITIS; RESPIRATORY AILMENTS; SKIN; FEMALE TONIC; BLOOD PURI/DETOX; CIRCULATION; FATIGUE; WEIGHT LOSS; ENVIRONMENTAL POLLUTION; FEVERS & INFECTIONS; THYROID; WHOLE BODY; DETOXIFY/NURTURE; MENTAL ALERTNESS/SENILITY)

KELP is used in Japan, China and Malaysia to treat uterine disorders, impotence and infertility, along with uterine disease and ovarian troubles. (**14**). Kelp's mode of action is probably derived from an extremely high content of trace minerals essential to proper hormone regulation by key glands and organs. (*See also CIRCULATION; THYROID; ENVIRONMENTAL POLLUTION; MENTAL ALERTNESS/SENILITY; PAIN; HEART; BLOOD PURI/DETOX; FATIGUE; WEIGHT LOSS; FEVERS & INFECTIONS*)

OTHER NUTRIENTS

VITAMINS
(Daily Requirements unless otherwise noted)
Vitamin A *25,000 I.U.*
Vitamin B Complex
Vitamin B1 *25-50 mg*
Vitamin C *1,000 - 3,000 mg.*
Vitamin E *up to 1600 I.U.*
Pantothenic Acid *50 - 100 mg*
Choline *1,000 mg*
Inositol *1,000 mg*
PABA *100 mg*
Folic Acid *up to 400 mcg*
Niacinamide *50 mg*

MINERALS
Iodine
Zinc
Calcium/Magnesium

MISCELLANEOUS
Brewer's yeast
Wheat Germ (oil)
Lecithin
Cod Liver Oil

REFERENCES

1. Roys, R.L. **The Ethno-Botany of the Maya**. Pub 2, Middle America Research Series, Tulane, University, New Orleans, 1931, p. 265.
2. Curtin, L.S.M. **Healing Herbs of the Upper Rio Grande**. Southwest Museum, Los Angeles, 1965.
3. Pearce, P.T., Zois, I., Wynne, K.N., Funder, J.W. "Panax Ginseng and Eleutherococcus senticosus extracts—in vitro studies on binding to steroid receptors." **Endocrinologica Japonica**, 1982, 29(5), 567-573.
4. Forgo, I., Kayasseh, L., Staub, J.J. "Effect of a standarized ginseng extract on general well being, reaction time, lung, function, and gonadal hormones." **Medizinische Welt**, 1981, 32(19), 751-756.
5. Culbreth, D.M.R. **A Manual of Materia Medica and Pharmacology**. Philadelphia, 1927, p. 99.
6. Potter, S.O.L. **Materia Medica, Pharmacy, and Therapeutics**. Philadelphia, 1906, 420.
7. Leung, A.Y. **Encyclopedia of Common Natural Ingredients**. New York, 1980, 152.
8. Kiangsu Institute of Modern Medicine. **Encyclopedia of Chinese Drugs**. 2 Vols, Shanghai, Peoples Republic of China, 1977.
9. Costello, C.H. & Lynn, E.V. "Estrogenic substances from plants: I. Glycyrrhiza glabra." **Journal of the American Pharmaceutical Association**, 39, 177-180, 1950.
10. Shiata, I. & Elghamry, M. "Estrogenic activity of glycyrrhiza glabra with its effect on uterine motility at various stages of the sex cycle." **Zentralblatt der Verterinarmedizin.**, Ser. A, 10, 155-162, 1963.
11. Sharaf, A., Gomaa, N. & El-Camal, M.H.A. "Glycyrrhetic acid as an active estrogenic substance separated from glycyrrhiza glabra (liquorice)." **Egyptian Journal of Pharmaceutical Sciences**, 16(2), 245-251, 1975.
12. Dekanski, J.B., Gottfried, S. & MacDonald, A. "Oestrogenic activity of enoxolone in rodents." **Journal of Pharmacy and Pharmacology**, 31, 62, 1979.
13. Yaginuma, T., Izumi, R., Yasui, H., Arai, T. & Kawabata, M. "Effect of traditional herbal medicine on serum testosterone levels and its induction of regular ovulation in hyper-androgenic and oligomenorrheic women." **Nippon Sanka Fujinka Gakkai Zasshi**, 1982, 34(7), 939-944.
14. Binding, G.J. & Moyle, A. **About Kelp**. Thorsons Publishers Limited. Wellingborough, Northamptonshire, England, 1974.

INFLUENZA

HERBS: GOLDENSEAL root (*Hydrastis canadensis*), BAYBERRY root bark (*Myrica cerifera*) Cayenne (*Capsicum annum*).

Form: Capsule.

PURPOSE: To help the body rid itself of infectious conditions such as Influenza (flu), colds, Sore throat, and Congestion.

Other Applications: None.

USE: 2-3 caps, 4 times per day throughout illness and convalescence. Supplement with 2-3 cap/day of FEVERS & INFECTIONS blend and 2-3 caps/day of RESPIRATORY AILMENTS to promote freer breathing.

Contraindications: None.

This is the blend to be using while you're suffering from common flus, colds, sore throats and so forth. It is essential to use this blend daily throughout the convalescence period to insure rapid and complete recovery and to lessen the chances of recurrent problems.

GOLDENSEAL ROOT acts on the nervous system very much like Cinchona. It is well-suited for treating the mucous membranes, especially in cases of vaginal and uterine infections. Goldenseal has found effective use as a restorative medication following protracted fevers. The alkaloids of Goldenseal, especially berberine and hydrastine, have been used to combat a wide variety of infectious agents (1-2). Goldenseal extract has been shown effective against staph, strep, tuberculosis and *escherichia coli (3-5)*. Goldenseal constituents have also been found to cure an increasingly troublesome, water-borne disease called giardiasis (6). (See also VAGINAL YEAST INFECTION; NERVES & GLANDS; STOMACH/INTESTINAL; EYES; FEVERS & INFECTIONS; HEMORRHOIDS)

BAYBERRY ROOT BARK contains antipyretic, antibiotic, and paramecicidal chemicals (7). Bayberry, an important nutritive supplement and digestive aid, helps insure that vital nutrients are absorbed into the blood stream. Bayberry root bark actually promotes healthy glandular activity throughout the entire body. Despite its widespread occurrence in North America, the Bayberry tree was used medicinally by just a few native American tribes. One group of Choctaws used it for fevers (8). (See also EYES)

CAYENNE increases the circulation of blood to peripheral tissues, ensuring that nutrients (including those obtained from this and other herbal preparations) are delivered to inflamed and infected areas. Though the practice is unsubstantiated scientifically, many people use Cayenne directly to treat sore throat and other cold symptoms, taking advantage of the herb's irritant property on the surface of exposed tissue. Others find this practice very painful, so exercise caution in applying the contents of these capsules directly to mucous membranes. (See also CIRCULATION; FATIGUE; HIGH BLOOD PRESSURE; BLOOD PURIFICATION/DETOXIFICATION)

OTHER NUTRIENTS

VITAMINS
(Daily requirements unless otherwise noted)

Vitamin A 25,000-50,000 I.U.	Vitamin C 3,000-5,000 mg
Vitamin B Complex	Vitamin D 400 I.U.
Vitamin B1 25-100 mg	Vitamin E 600 I.U.
Vitamin B2 25-100 mg	Pantothenic Acid 50 mg
Vitamin B6 25-100 mg	Niacinamide 50 mg

MINERALS
Calcium/Magnesium
Phosphorous
Potassium
Sodium

MISCELLANEOUS
Cod Liver Oil
Essential Fatty Acid
GLA
HCl

REFERENCES

1. Kulkarni, S.K., Dandiya, P.C. & Varandani, N.L. "Pharmacological investigations of berberine sulphate." **JapanMrq Journal of Pharmacology**, 22, 11-16, 1972.
2. Dutta, N.K. & Panse, M.V. "Usefulness of berberine in the treatment of cholera." **Indian Journal of Medical Research**, 50(5), 732-736, 1962.
3. D'Amico, M.L. "Ricerche sulla presenza di sostanze ad azione antibiotica nelle piante superiori." **Fitoterapia**, 21(1), 77-79, 1950.
4. Orzechowski, G. "Antibiotics from higher plants." **Pharmazie in unserer Zeit**, 10, 42-54, 1981.
5. Fitzpatrick, F.K. "Plant substances active against mycobacterium tuberculosis." **Antibiotics and Chemotherapy**, 4(5), 528-536, 1954.
6. Gupte, S. "Use of berberine in treatment of giardiasis." **American Journal of Diseases of Childhood**, 129, 866, 1975.
7. Paul, B.D., Rao, G.S. & Kapaida, G.J. "Isolation of myricadiol, myricitrin, taraxerol, and taraxerone from myrica cerifera root bark." **Journal of Pharmaceutical Science**, 63(6), 958-959, 1974.
8. Bushnell, D.I., Jr. **The Choctaw of Bayou Lacomb, St. Tammany Parish, Louisiana.** Bureau of American Ethnology Bulletin Nr. 48, Washington D.C., Government Printing Office, 1909.

INSOMNIA

HERBS: VALERIAN root (*Valeriana officinalis*), HOPS (*Humulus lupulus*), Skullcap (*Scutellaria lateriflora*), & Passion Flower (*Passiflora incarnata*).

Form: Capsule.

PURPOSE: To overcome common sleep disorders and nervous disorders; sedation.

Other Applications: Anxiety, restlessness, hyperactivity, to relax, to aid meditation.

USE: 1. Insomnia: 2 caps one hour before retiring; 2 caps upon retiring.
2. Nervous disorders: 2 caps, 3 times per day or as needed.
3. For relaxation or sedation: 2-4 caps as needed.

Contraindications: None. Do not use while driving.

Although insomnia is not well understood, most experts agree that in 95% of the cases insomnia is a side effect or symptom rather than a primary disease in and of itself. Emotional stress, anxiety, and pain are common causes of insomnia. One of my earliest research projects on herbs involved observing the effects of a blend containing Valerian root, Skullcap and Hops, on a woman who had suffered, by her report, insomnia and other sleep disorders before she began using that blend and still suffered whenever she forgot to take it. The results showed that she slept longer and got to sleep faster, and felt better in the morning when she took the "real" blend. Passion Flower adds another proven sedative principle.

VALERIAN ROOT is a primary sedative and is used when sleep disorders are the result of anxiety, nervousness, exhaustion, headache or hysteria. See the chapter on NERVOUS TENSION for a discussion of this herb's sedative properties. Valerian root has been used for these purposes since pre-Christian times and is cited in virtually every pharmacopoeia in the world. It is not surprising that modern science has confirmed its actions experimentally. (See also HIGH BLOOD PRESSURE; NERVOUS TENSION)

HOPS, like Valerian root, also have pronounced sedative effects (1). Taken internally, remarkably large amounts of Hops can be used without fear of any side effects. The active principle of Hops is normally assumed to be lupulin, but recent research suggests that other constituents may be even more important (2). (See also NERVOUS TENSION)

SKULLCAP is another favorite remedy for sleep disorders and nervous complaints of all types. It occurs in this blend in greater concentration than in the NERVOUS TENSION blend, so that its ability to induce sleep is felt in greater measure. It is especially effective in reducing the severity of pain that sometimes accompanies sleep, and it numbs pains and aches that prevent some individuals from falling asleep easily. (See also PAIN RELIEF; NERVOUS TENSION; NERVES & GLANDS)

PASSION FLOWER is an extremely popular herb in Europe where it is often used to induce relaxation and sleep (3), an effect first experimentally verified in 1920 (4). In that study, the researcher noticed that, unlike what happens with narcotics, sleep was induced normally, with easy, light breathing, with little or no neural or mental depression. Upon awakening the patients showed no signs of confusion or stupor or melancholy. In 1979, about 50 preparations on the market in Germany contained Passion Flower. Forty two were sedatives and 6 were cardiotonics. These preparations were recommended for the following conditions: 1. Nervous or easily aroused children; 2. Cardiovascular neurosis; 3. Bronchial asthma; 4. Coronary diseases; 5. Weak circulation; 6. Sleep disorders; 7. Problems of concentration in school children; and 8. Geriatrics (7). (See also NERVOUS TENSION; FEMALE TONIC)

OTHER NUTRIENTS

VITAMINS
(Daily requirements unless otherwise noted)

Vitamin B-1 25-100 mg	Vitamin D 400 mg
Vitamin B-2 25-100 mg	Vitamin E 400-600 mg
Vitamin B-6 25-100 mg	Niacinamide 100 mg
Vitamin C 500 mg	Pantothenic Acid 150-200 mg

MINERALS
Calcium/Magnesium

MISCELLANEOUS
Potassium

REFERENCES

1. Wohlfart, R., Haensel, R. & Schmidt, H. "The sedative-hypnotic principle of hops (4)." **Planta Medica**, 48, 120-123, 1983.
2. Wohlfart, R., Haensel, R. & Schmidt, H. "An investigation of sedative-hypnotic principles in Hops. Part 3." **Planta Medica**, 45, 224, 1982.
3. Lutomski, J. "Alkaloidy passiflora incarnata I." **Diss. Institut fuer Heilpflanzenforschung**, Poznan, 1960.4. Lutomski, J., Segiet, E., Szpunar, K. & Grisse, K. "The meaning of Passion Flower in the healing arts." **Pharmazie in Unserer Zeit**, 10(2), 45-49, 1981.

LAXATIVE

HERBS: BUTTERNUT root bark (*Juglans cinera*), **CASCARA** Sagrada bark (*Rhamnus purshiana*), **Rhubarb root** (*Rheum palmatum*), **Ginger root** (*Zingiber officinale*), **Licorice root** (*Glycyrrhiza glabra*), **Irish Moss** (*Chondrus crispus*), & **Cayenne** (*Capsicum annum*).

Form: Capsule.

PURPOSE: Laxative. Gentle but effective.

Other Applications: To treat G.I. bleeding (1). As an adjunct in the treatment of liver disorders.

USE: Children under 5: Not recommended. Use bulk laxatives, such as Psyllium seed. Children over 5: One cap every 8 hours. Youth, 13-17: 2-3 caps every 8 hours. Youth, 16-21: 2-3 caps every 6 hours. Adults under 60: 2-3 caps every 4 hours. Adults over 60: 1-2 caps every 8 hours. NOTE: One may expect considerable variation in these recommendations, depending upon general health, diet and medications being used.

Contraindications: None.

Constipation may be chronic, acute or simple diet-induced irregularity. Proper cathartic (an agent that promotes intestinal evacuation) treatment regimens for both chronic and acute constipation are built around the sensible use of several herbs. The proper treatment for diet-induced constipation is to include prunes, bran- and fiber-containing foods in the diet, and to cut out drugs such as caffeine and alcohol. It should be noted here that chronic constipation is often the result of the abuse of cathartics themselves. If you belong to the group of individuals who habitually use carthartics to induce bowel movements, you may be able to help your body regain control over this process by using only mild cathartics such as those in this blend, learning to relax and not worry about your condition, and by changing your dietary habits to include bran and fiber. Expect emotional strains and tensions as you begin to turn control of your bowel back to your body.

BUTTERNUT ROOT BARK, during the last century, was known as one of the "most mild and efficacious laxatives" (1), as one of of the "best and safest" laxatives to be found (2). We are witnessing in this century a well-deserved renewal of interest in the cathartic properties of this herb. Butternut root bark is good not only as a laxative but as a treatment for liver disorders and intestinal sickness (as practiced extensively in homeopathy). *(See also FEVERS & INFECTIONS)*

CASCARA SAGRADA bark, dried and cured, is one of the most effective, gentle and non-habituating laxatives available. It is used very often not only by herbalists, but by doctors and the general public as well. Many proprietary laxatives are built around Cascara. Its effectiveness is mainly due to its high anthraquinone content (3-4). Anthraquinones, or A-factors produce a soft or formed stool in about six to eight hours with little or no griping. The 1977 Formulary Service of the American Society of Hospital Pharmacists, Inc., emphasizes the mild action of Cascara and remarks further that the herb does not lose its efficiency with repeated use. In fact, Cascara can be used to correct the habitual constipation incurred by the abuse of other laxatives. Many over-the-counter laxatives contain Cascara, but you must be careful which one you pick, because some contain substances of questionable value, such as belladonna alkaloids, podophyllum, aloin and strychnine. Summarizing the beneficial properties of Cascara, we note that: 1) the cathartic action is mild; 2) it is **un**accompanied by discomfort, griping or colic; 3) its action is limited to the large bowel; 4) its efficiency is not lost with repeated use; 5) it is not habit forming; and 6) it can correct habitual constipation by restoring intestinal tonus. *(See also DETOXIFY/NURTURE; LIVER DISORDERS)*

RHUBARB, cultivated in China and Tibet, has an illustrious history of inclusion in many laxative preparations. It is generally considered a mild laxative that produces a soft stool 6-10 hours after ingestion (5), but should not be used by itself when the colon is totally evacuated, because the presence of astringent tannins may produce constipative feelings. On very rare occasions sensitive persons may experience mild colicky pains. The herb is an important part of this blend because the A-factors of the herb differ somewhat from those of Cascara. Only some of them reach the large intestines intact, while others are resorbed in the small intestine and are later released into the large intestine (6). The timing of the activity of Rhubarb is thus displaced to some degree from the other laxative agents in this blend, thereby promoting longer and smoother activity of the whole. Rhubarb is especially well suited for children since is very mild in action. For chronic constipation, it may be used year-round, but should only be given when necessary, since prolonged use may lead to potassium deficiency. Rhubarb is, therefore, best used in a blend that respects the functioning of the whole organism.

GINGER ROOT plays an important role in this blend; namely, it counterbalances the discomforting effects of colon reflex activity and imparts a pleasant degree of mildness to the blend's functioning. Ginger root also helps restore and normalize proper tone and reflex faculty to the gastro-intestinal tract (7). It is not only important that one use a proper laxative, but that one revitalize sick and flaccid muscles and glands. Ginger root helps do this. In addition, Ginger root has been shown to normalize peristalsis (8). *(See also DIGESTION; STOMACH/INTESTINAL; NAUSEA; FATIGUE; LOW BLOOD SUGAR; CIRCULATION)*

LICORICE ROOT, besides being a mild aperient itself, helps to counterbalance the discomforting effects that may result from laxative use. It provides a mild boost to the adrenal system that may be stressed in certain debilitating conditions for which laxatives are often suggested. Most importantly Licorice root protects and heals distressed mucous membranes of the intestinal tract as confirmed by literally hundreds of studies (e.g., 9). *(See also INFERTILITY; ARTHRITIS; RESPIRATORY AILMENTS; SKIN DISORDERS; FEMALE TONIC; BLOOD PURI/DETOX; CIRCULATION; FATIGUE; WEIGHT LOSS; ENVIR POLLU; FEVERS & INFECTIONS; THYROID; WHOLE BODY; DETOX/NURTURE; MENTAL ALERT/SENILITY)*

IRISH MOSS is used as a stabilizer in such dairy products as ice creams, sherbets, chocolate milk, yogurt and whipped creams. It is used in syrups and toppings and provides both mouth feel and body to creamed soups and chowders. Since it is an unassimilated hydrocolloid it is used in raw form as a bulk laxative. It also coats and soothes the entire gastrointestinal tract. In various forms, it alleviates peptic and duodenal ulcers in humans while having no adverse effects on the colon (10). *(See also STOMACH/INTESTINAL; THYROID)*

CAYENNE provides just a little zip to the blend, acting as it does in so many cases, as an effective catalyst and augmenter of the other principles in the blend.

OTHER NUTRIENTS

VITAMINS
(Daily requirements unless otherwise noted)
- Vitamin A *25,000 I.U.*
- Vitamin B-1 *25-100 mg*
- Vitamin B-2 *25-100 mg*
- Vitamin B-6 *25-100 mg*
- Vitamin C *500-1000 mg*
- Vitamin D *400 I.U.*
- Vitamin E *200 I.U.*
- Niacinamide *50 mg*
- Choline *300-500 mg*
- Inositol *200-400 mg*

MINERALS
- Potassium
- Calcium/Magnesium

MISCELLANEOUS
- Bran
- Fiber
- Prunes

REFERENCES

1. Bigelow, J. **American Medical Botany, Being a Collection of the Native Medicinal Plants of the United States.** 3 vols. Cummings & Hilliard, Boston, 1817-1820.
2. Gunn, J.D. **New Domestic Physician or Home Book of Health.** Moore, Wilstach, Keys. 686, 1971. Cincinnati, 1st ed., 1857 and 1861 edition.
3. Nelemans, F.A. **Pharmacology.** 14, suppl. I, 73-77, 1976.
4. Godding, E.W. **Pharmacology.** 14, Suppl. 1, 78-101, 1976.
5. List, P.H. & Hoerhammer, L. **Hagers Handbuch der Pharmazeutischen Praxis.** Volumes 2-5, Springer-Verlag, Berlin.
6. Chirikdjian, J.J., Kopp, B. & Beran, H. "Laxative action of a new anthraquinone glycoside from rhubarb root." **Planta Medica**, 48(1), 34-37, 1983.
7. Glatzel, H. "Treatment of dyspeptic disorders with spice extracts." **Hippocrates**, 40(23), 916-919, 1969.
8. Glatzel, H. **Dtsh Apoth Ztg,** 110, 5, 1970.
9. Cooke, W.M. & Baron, J.H. "Metabolic studies of deglycyrrhizinised licorice in two patients with gastric ulcers." **Digestion**, 4, 264-268, 1971.
10. **Martindale: The Extra Pharmacopoeia.** 1977. The Pharmaceutical Press. London.

LIVER DISORDERS

HERBS: DANDELION root (*Taraxacum officinale*), CASCARA Sagrada bark, (*Rhamnus purshiana*) Licorice root (*Glycyrrhiza glabra*), Celery seed (*Apium graveolens*), Cayenne (*Capsicum annum*), Wild Yam root (*Dioscorea villosa*).

Form: Capsule.

PURPOSE: To assist the body remedy liver disorders (hepatitis, cirrhosis and jaundice); Also maintains healthy liver, gallbladder, pancreas, and spleen; laxative.

Other Applications: Colon stimulant, indigestion and heartburn, gastritis, gallstones, constipation.

USE: 1. Hepatitis, cirrhosis, jaundice: 4-6 caps/day, plus 2-3 caps of the FEVERS & INFECTIONS Blend.
  2. For gallbladder problems: 2-4 caps/day along with 2-4 caps of the FEVERS & INFECTIONS blend.
  3. For glandular maintenance: 4-5 caps/day. May use along with the TONIC—NERVE & GLAND blend.
  4. Supplement with BLOOD PURI/DETOX Blend.

Contraindications: Though no evidence exists to prove that the steroid precursors in Wild Yam are allergenic, persons with severe estrogenic sensitivity should exercise caution if exceeding 2-4 capsules per day.

Close to two dozen major functions are performed by the liver on a continuous basis. In order to perform all of these functions, the liver processes an incredible amount of blood, about three pints every minute. When the liver is diseased, many of these functions do not operate correctly. Toxins are no longer filtered out efficiently and may build up in the body, as will the the by-products of protein metabolism such as ammonia. Sugar levels fall. Infection is common, and the kidneys may fail. Severe, uncontrollable bleeding is also common, with coma and death likely. But checked in time, a diseased or failed liver stands a good chance of healing very well. You may notice a strong similarity between this blend and the DIABETES blend. Dandelion heads up the list of ingredients in both; however, the primary purpose of this product is to aid the body in combating various liver-related problems. The blend contains herbs with extremely effective principles and should prove to be one of the most effective blends in this book.

DANDELION ROOT heads the list of excellent medicinal foods for the liver and related organs and glands. This high position is supported by available research. It stimulates the flow of bile directly (**1**), and promotes the flow of bile by inducing contraction of the gallbladder (**2**). Dandelion dramatically improves such conditions as bile duct inflammation, liver congestion and gall stones (**2**), and has been used to treat chronic hepatitis, swelling of the liver, jaundice and dyspepsia with deficient bile secretion (**3**). *(See also DIABETES; BLOOD PURI/DETOX; SKIN DISORDERS; NERVES & GLANDS)*

CASCARA SAGRADA, normally a great laxative, is used in smaller amounts in folk medicine to treat liver disorders and gallstones. Its use to remedy hepatic disease has been confirmed by modern research (**5**). *(See also DETOXIFY/NURTURE; LAXATIVE)*

LICORICE ROOT as a treatment for hepatitis is thought to have originated in China. In Europe, Licorice root, because of its mild diuretic property, is used to treat urinary and kidney problems. Licorice root decreases the accumulation of triglyceride in the liver, increases glycogen levels, prevents the development of experimental cirrhosis and prevents the occurrence of experimentally induced lesions in the liver (**7**). In Japan, a popular preparation composed of glycyrrhizin (an active constituent of Licorice root) has been extensively used to treat hepatitis with a great deal of success (**8**). While nobody is certain how it works, a recent study found that Licorice root induces the production of interferon, a substance produced by the body that is successfully used to treat victims of hepatitis B (**8**). *(See also INFERTILITY; ARTHRITIS; THYROID; WHOLE BODY; SKIN DISORDERS; RESPIRATORY AILMENTS; FEMALE TONIC; CIRCULATION; WEIGHT LOSS; ENVIRONMENTAL POLLUTION; MENTAL ALERTNESS/SENILITY; DETOXIFY/NURTURE; FEVERS & INFECTIONS)*

CELERY SEED has not been subjected to the same amount of research investigation as many other herbs. Nevertheless, in addition to its diuretic activity, it has been shown to possess other definite medicinal properties, including insulin-like activity (**9**) and the ability to suppress adrenaline hyperglycemia (**10**). These findings suggest that this lowly herb, if eaten regularly, can promote a certain degree of health in the vital organs of the body. *(See also ARTHRITIS)*

CAYENNE again acts as the catalyst and reaction promoter in this blend, enhancing its overall effectiveness.

WILD YAM ROOT preparations were used to treat bilious colic by American physicians long before the herb's steroid properties became known. It sometimes rapidly and effectively reduced the pain of biliary colic, caused by gallstones; and eased the passage of **small** stones (**6**). Some writers noted that the treatment did not always work, but that it was nevertheless one of the best antispasmotic treatments known, applicable for all forms of colicky and paroxysmal pain, ovarian neuralgia, spasmotic dysmenorrhea and indigestion (**4**). Part of the therapeutic action of Wild Yam root on overall liver health is due to its ability to lower blood cholesterol levels and lower blood pressure. These properties would indirectly help the liver by increasing its efficiency and reducing stress (**11**). *(See also FEMALE TONIC)*

OTHER NUTRIENTS

VITAMINS
(Daily requirements unless otherwise noted)
  Vitamin A *25,000-50,000 I.U.*
  Vitamin B1 *25-100 mg*
  Vitamin B2 *25-100 mg*
  Vitamin B6 *25-100 mg*
  Vitamin C *1,000-10,000 mg*
  Vitamin D *400 I.U.*
  Vitamin E *400-600 I.U.*
  Choline *2-3 g*
  Inositol *2-3 g*
  Folic acid *40 mcg*

MINERALS

MISCELLANEOUS
  Brewer's Yeast
  Lecithin
  Yogurt
  Liver
  Protein

REFERENCES

1. Buesemaker, "Concerning the choleretic activity of Dandelion," **Naunyn-Schmiederbergs Archiv fuer Experimentelle Pharmakology und Pathologie**, 181, 512, 1936.
2. Leclerc, H. **Phytotherapie**, Paris, 1927, cited by Ripperger, W. "Pflanzliche laxantien und cholagogue wirkungen." **Med Welt**, 9, 1463-1467, 1935.
3. Bentely, R. & Trimen, H. **Medicinal Plants**, J & A Churchill, London, 1880, Vol 3, 159.
4. Felter, H. W. **The Eclectic Materia Medica, Pharmacology and Therapeutics.** Eclectic Medical Publications, Portland, Oregon, 1983 (first published 1922).
5. Kerharo, J. & Bouquet, A. **Plantes Medicinales et Toxiques de la Cole d'Ivoire**, Haute-Vota, Vigot, Paris, 1950.
6. Ellingwood, F. **American Materia Medica, Therapeutics and Pharmacognosy.** Eclectic Medical Publications, Portland, Oregon, 1983.
7. Zhao, M., Han, D., Ma, X., Zhao, Y., Yin, L. & Li, C. "The preventive and therapeutic actions of glycyrrhizin, glycyrrhetic acid and crude saikosides on experimental cirrhosis in rats." **Yao Hsueh Hsueh Pao**, 18(5), 325-331, 1983.
8. Fujisawa, K., Watanabe, Y. & Kimura, K. "Therapeutic approach to chronic active hepatitis with glycyrrhizin." **Asian Medical Journal**, 23, 745-756, 1980.
9. Best, C.H. & Scott, D.A. "Possible sources of insulin." **Journal of Metabolic Research**, 3, 177-179, 1923.
10. Sharaf, A.A., Hussein, A.M. & Mansour, M.Y. "Studies on the antidiabetic effect of some plants." **Planta Medica**, 2, 159-168, 1963.
11. Sokolova, L.H. "Effect of saponins on the development of experimental atherosclerosis." **Farmakologia i Toxikologia**, 21(6), 85-90, 1958.

MENSTRUATION

HERBS: **CRANESBILL** root (*Geranium maculatum*), **RASPBERRY** leaves (*Rubus idaeus*), **Witch Hazel leaves** (*Hamamelis virginiana*), **Uva-Ursi leaves** (*Arctostaphylos uva-ursi*), **Papaya leaves** (*Carica papaya*), **Shepherd's Purse** (*Capsella bursa-pastoris*), **Black Haw bark** (*Viburnum prunifolium*).

Form: Capsule, Douche, Enema, Tea, Gargle

PURPOSE: To decrease excessive flow during menstruation. Astringent.

Other Applications: To be used externally or internally, wherever there is a need for a powerful astringent: Hemorrhage; internal bleeding caused by ulcers; diarrhea; hemorrhoids; chronic mucous discharges.

USE: 1. Menorrhagia (excessive menstrual flow): 4-6 caps/day. Tea: 4 caps; Douche: From cool tea; Enema: From warm tea.
2. Hemorrhoids: Use with HEMORRHOIDS Blend: 3 each/day.
3. To supplement the VAGINAL YEAST INFECTION Blend: 2-3 caps/day, or 2 caps/meal.

Contraindications: None.

Excessive menstrual flow may signal the presence of mild to severe underlying disease, even cancer, and must be brought to your physician's attention. Meanwhile, you should be aware that iron is being lost and must be replaced. Iodine and Vitamin C must also be replenished regularly. This blend can and should be used by anybody in need of astringent medication. It extends and amplifies the astringent principle found in the VAGINAL YEAST INFECTION blend. Its purpose is to rapidly correct many forms of diarrhea, and to ameliorate symptoms of slow, steady menorrhagia.

CRANESBILL ROOT was relied upon by early American Indians to treat diarrhea, dysentery, leukorrhea, and hemorrhoids, among other conditions. These people passed this knowledge on to the early settlers, and thus into the black bag of many early physicians, who discovered it would also reduce chronic menorrhagia (1), especially in cases of prolonged, but slow bleeding. One early physician remarked, "I ...esteem geranium (cranesbill) more highly than any other vegetable astringent, where a simple tonic astringent action is needed. It is palatable, prompt, efficient, and invariable in its effects, and entirely devoid of unpleasant influences," (2).

WITCH HAZEL LEAF appears in this blend, as well as VAGINAL YEAST INFECTION, because of its reliable astringent property. The reader is referred to the V.Y.I. blend for a discussion, and to the HEMORRHOIDS/ASTRINGENT Blend for a discussion of Witch Hazel's involvement in hemorrhoid treatment.

RASPBERRY LEAF provides adjunctive support for the anti-diarrheal aspect of this blend. That effect is primarily due to the astringent nature of the leaves. In addition, Raspberry leaves are important to some of the secondary applications of this product. One scientific study showed that a principle in the leaf is responsible for relaxing the smooth muscles of the uterus and intestine when they are in tone, and that same principle causes contraction of the uterus when it is not in tone (3). The relaxation effect probably accounts for the traditional therapeutic value of Raspberry leaves in aiding parturition. The contracting effect may explain the ability of the leaves to remedy extreme laxity of the bowels. *(See also FEMALE TONIC; DIABETES; EYES)*

UVA-URSI LEAF, is a confirmed astringent with urinary antiseptic properties (4). This action is due to the high concentration of a known antiseptic, arbutin, in the herb. Arbutin, in passing through the system, yields hydroquinone, which may turn the urine dark or brownish-green, a harmless condition. Hydroquinone is a urinary disinfectant. Uva-ursi leaves also contain anesthetic principles capable of numbing pain in the urinary system. *(See also DIURETIC; DIABETES)*

PAPAYA LEAF is best known as a digestive aid, but is included in this blend on the strength of recent research findings that indicate that it also possesses an antihemolytic property, i.e., it should reduce the severity of bleeding and hemorrhage throughout the body (6). In this regard, it will inhibit menorrhagia. It is also an emmenagogue, that is, it will promote menstruation in women who have trouble menstruating, or who menstruate only with pain. *(See also DIGESTION; STOMACH/INTESTINAL)*

SHEPHERD'S PURSE possesses mild astringency. It also contains several substances which could help female physiological processes. It is effective in treating menorrhagia characterized by lengthy and frequent almost colorless flow (2). Basic chemical analysis has determined that the principles of Shepherd's Purse coagulate blood (7). The herb also reduces urinary tract irritation and atony. It will clear up blood in the urine, and may eliminate mild forms of hemorrhage. Studies have found a uterine contracting property in Shepherd's Purse (8). And the herb has also been found to enhance uterine tonus (5).

BLACK HAW BARK was a discovery of the early American physician, who used it more than any other herb for practically all female problems, believing it would relax the uterus, relieve painful menstruation, fight diarrhea, and generally tone up the whole female reproductive system (9). Use of the herb tapered off during the 1st half of this century, but Black Haw is now enjoying a comeback. Recently, chemists discovered several uterine muscle relaxants in the herb (10).

OTHER NUTRIENTS

VITAMINS
(Daily requirements unless otherwise noted)
Vitamin A *25,000 I.U.*
Vitamin B1 *25-50 mg*
Vitamin B2 *25-50mg*
Vitamin B6 *25-50mg*
Vitamin B12 *up to 50 mcg*
Vitamin C *1000 mg*
Vitamin D *400 I.U.*
Vitamin E *600 I.U.*
Folic Acid *400 mcg*

MINERALS
Iron
Iodine
Calcium/Magnesium

REFERENCES

1. Felter, H.W. **The Eclectic Materia Medica, Pharmacology and Therapeutics.** Eclectic Medical Pubs, Portland, 1983, 391 (1st published, 1922).
2. Ellingwood, R. **American Materia Medica, Therapeutics and Pharmacognosy.** Eclectic Medical Pub., Portland, 1983. 347.
3. Burn, J.H. & Withell, E.R. "A principle in raspberry leaves which relaxes uterine muscles." **Lancet.** 2(6149), 1-3, 1941.
4. List, P.H. & Hoerhammer, L. **Hagers Handbuch der Pharmazeutischen Praxis.** vols 2-5. Springer-Verlag. Berlin. 1969-1976.
5. Trease, G.E. & Evans, W.C. **Pharmacognosy.** 1978. 11th ed. Bailliere Tindall. London.
6. Pousset, J.L. "Antihemolytic action of an extract of Carica papaya bark. Possibilities of use in glucose-6-phosphate dehydrogenase deficiencies." **Dakar Med,** 1979, 24(3), 255-262.
7. Kuroda, K. & Takagi, K. "Physiologically active substances in capsella bursa pastoris." **Nature,** 220(5168), 707-708, 1968.
8. Kuroda, K. & Kaku, T. "Pharmacological and chemical studies on the alcohol extract of capsella bursa pastoris." **Life Sciences,** 8(3), 151-155, 1969.
9. Hale, E.M. **The Special Symptomatology of the New Remedies.** Philadelphia, 1877.
10. Jarboe, C.H., Schmidt, C.M. & Nicholson, J.A. & Zirvi, K.A. "Uterine relaxant properties of viburnum." **Nature.** 212, 837, 1966

MENTAL ALERTNESS/SENILITY

HERBS: PEPPERMINT (*Mentha piperita*), **SIBERIAN GINSENG** (*Eleutherococcus senticosus*), **Skullcap** (*Scutellaria lateriflora*), **Wood Betony** (*Stachys officinalis*), **Gotu Kola** (*Hydrocotyle asiatica*), & **Kelp** (*Laminaria, Macrocystis, Ascophyllum*).

Form: Capsule, Tea

PURPOSE: To improve poor memory; To increase concentration capability and mental stamina; to overcome the effects of aging on mental attributes.

Other Applications: Poor circulation, irritability, anxiety, insomnia, hyperactivity, depression.

USE: 1. Adults, general use: As desired, up to 12 caps/day.
2. Adults, acute conditions: 3-4 caps, 3 times/day.
3. Hyperactive children: 2-3 capsin morning; 1-2 caps at Dinner. Use 3-4 caps of Ginger root per day.

Contraindications: None.

The goals of this blend are to help younger, healthy individuals improve the efficiency of their mental faculties, to prevent the onset of senile brain damage, to arrest any degeneration in progress, or delay its onset as long as possible, to help healthy tissue compensate for deficiencies, and secondarily, to curb irritability, hypersensitivity, etc. To accomplish these ends the blend must increase healthy arterial and venous circulation, and improve the general health of the nervous system and the rest of the body, especially the adrenal system. These herbs provide circulation to the cells of the brain, nurture nerves, calm irritability, impart restfulness and clarity of mind, and generally increase mental capabilities.

PEPPERMINT LEAF, due to the presence of several essential oils, prevents congestion of the blood supply to the brain, helps to clear up any circulatory congestion that exists, stimulates circulation, and strengthens and calms nerves. University students have benefited greatly through participation in loosely controlled experiments assessing the effects of Peppermint tea on test-taking skills and examination scores (**1**). *(See also FATIGUE; DIGESTION)*

SIBERIAN GINSENG is, of course, the famous Asiatic tonic, that has been shown in numerous studies to affect mental and physical behavior (e.g., **2**). In geriatric use, Ginseng has been proven beneficial in restoring mental abilities (**3**). Ginseng helps by directly affecting the adrenal-pituitary axis (**4**), which effect is most often manifested as increased resistance to the effects of stress (**5**). The herb also aids mental function by improving circulation (**6**). Animal studies have also demonstrated the ability of Ginseng to help learning (**7**). Other studies show that Ginseng is a direct central nervous system stimulant (**8**). *(See also FATIGUE; WHOLE BODY; INFERTILITY; LOW BLOOD SUGAR)*

SKULLCAP is one of the best nervines in the plant kingdom. Read about this herb in the chapters on INSOMNIA, NERVOUS TENSION, NERVES & GLANDS and PAIN RELIEF. We note here only that the herb probably affects mental abilities by removing the nervous tension that often interferes with learning, recall, logical thinking and memory formation. In this regard, it very much resembles a muscle relaxant (**9**).

WOOD BETONY is also a good nervine with known hypotensive properties (**10**). It is used primarily to reduce nervousness through a mild sedative action. *(See also INSOMNIA; NERVOUS TENSION; PAIN RELIEF)*

GOTU KOLA, being a naturally excellent neural tonic, slowly builds mental stamina and neural health. It is an excellent treatment for nervous breakdown. In addition, Gotu Kola, according to Asian and European practice, is an excellent blood purifier, glandular tonic and diuretic. The people of India use the plant specifically to improve memory and longevity (**11**). *(See also FATIGUE; WHOLE BODY TONIC)*

KELP is included in this blend to provide nutritional support to the nervous system and heart, in the form of vitamins, minerals and cell salts. In addition, it supplies hypotensive and serum cholesterol lowering principles which are likely to have a sparing effect on cardiac and neural tissues by saving them from unnecessary stress, by prolonging their effective lifetime, and increasing their efficiency during daily use (**12-14**). *(See also FEVERS & INFECTIONS; CIRCULATION; THYROID; ENVIRONMENTAL POLLUTION; PAIN; INFERTILITY; HEART; FATIGUE; BLOOD PURI/DETOX; WEIGHT LOSS)*

OTHER NUTRIENTS

VITAMINS
(Daily requirements unless otherwise noted)
Vitamin B ComplexVitamin B1 *25-300 mg*
Vitamin B2 *25-300 mg*
Vitamin B6 *25-300 mg*
Vitamin C *1,000-3,000 mg*
Vitamin E *400 I.U.*
Choline *1,000 mg.*
Inositol *1,000 mg*
Folic Acid *400 mcg*
Niacinamide *100 mg*

MINERALS
Calcium/Magnesium
Phosphorous
Zinc

MISCELLANEOUS
HCl
Brewer's yeast

REFERENCES

1. Mowrey, D.B. Informal study conducted among graduate students at Brigham Young University, 1978. Was not double-blind, but did include a placebo control group.
2. Takagi, K. "Pharmacological studies of some oriental medicinals." **Yakhak Hoe Chi**, 17(1), 1-8, 1973.
3. Zhou, D.H. "preventive geriatrics: an overview from traditional chinese medicine." **American Journal of Chinese Medicine**, 10(1-4), 32-39, 1982.
4. Hai, S., Yokoyama, H., Oura, H. & Yano, S. "Stimulation of pituitary-adrenocortical system by ginseng saponins." **Endocrinologica Japonica**, 26(6), 661-665, 1979.
5. Freidman, S.L. & Khlebnikov, A.N. **Biologicheski Aktivnye Veshchestva (Mikroelementy, Vitaminy i Drugie) v Rastenievodstve Zhivotnovodstve i Meditsin.**, 113-116, 1975.
6. Kehara, M., Shibata, Y., Higashi, et. al. "Effect of ginseng saponins on cholesterol metabolism. III. Effect of ginsenoside-Rb on cholesterol synthesis in rats fed on high fat diet." **Chemical and Pharmaceutical Bulletin**, (Tokyo), 26(9), 2844-2854.
7. Saito, H., Tsuchiya, M., Naka, S. & Takagi, K. "Effects of Panax Ginseng root on acquisition of sound discrimination behavaior in rats." **Japanese Journal of Pharmacology**, 29, 319-324, 1979.
8. Petkov, V.W. "About the method of operation of Panax ginseng." **Arzneimittel-Forschung**, 11, 288-295, 1961.
9. Usow, V. **Farmakologiia I Toksikologiia**, 21(2), 31-34, 1958.
10. Zinchenko, T.V. & Fefer, I.M. "Investigation of glycosides from betonica officinalis." **Farmatsevt. Zhurnal**, 17(3), 35-38, 1962.
11. Chopra, R.N. **Indigenous Drugs of India**. Arts Press, Calcutta, 2nd Ed., Chopra, R.N., Chopra, I.C.,et al., Calcutta, India, 1933.
12. Kameda, J. "Medical studies on seaweeds. I." **Fukushima Igaku Zasshi**, 10, 251-269, 1960.
13. Kameda, J. "Medical studies on seaweeds. II." **Fukushima Igaku Zasshi**, 11, 289-309, 1961.
14. Ozawa, H., Gomi, Y. & Otsuki, I. "Pharmacological studies on laminine monocitrate." **Yakugaku Zasshi**, 87(8), 935-939, 1967.

NAUSEA

HERBS: **GINGER** root (*Zingiber officinale*), **Licorice root** (*Glycyrrhiza glabra*), & **Cayenne**, (*Capsicum annuum*).

Form: Capsule

PURPOSE: To help diminish the symptoms of nausea that result from motion sickness, morning sickness, or stomach disorders; to ameliorate symptoms of vertigo and dizziness.

Other Applications: Headaches; Learning disabilities that result from inner ear disturbances.

USE: 1. Nausea: The use of this blend to treat nausea is somewhat unique among herbal preparations. The basic rule ofthumb is "Use enough that you experience a Ginger aftertaste like a mild burning sensation in the throat and/or stomach." That might be two capsules, like before a road, plane or boat trip, or a dozen capsules, as during a case of stomach flu. The following are rough guides:

Motion Sickness: 2-4 caps 1/2 hour ahead of time; 2-4 caps whenever symptoms first begin to occur

Morning Sickness: 3-8 caps before arising; 3-5 caps as needed

Dizziness, Vertigo: 2 caps every 1/2 hour

Stomach Flu: 4-6 caps at first indication; As many as needed every 1/2 hour from then on.

Headache: 2-4 caps as needed.

Contraindications: None. Only minute amounts of Licorice and Cayenne should be in this blend. Their influence should only be felt when large quantities of the blend are being ingested, and then the influence will only be mild.

Nausea is a symptom that arises from many physiological conditions, some of which are the result of stomach and digestive problems, such as the flu, gallstones, indigestion and poisoning. Conditions like ear infections, vertigo, motion sickness, headache, fever and inflammations, psychological stimuli, and dizziness cause nausea indirectly, taking advantage of rich neural connections between the stomach and certain brain centers. Certain nutritional states, such as pantothenic acid and vitamin B6 deficiencies, can make a person more susceptible than usual to nausea-causing events. Most medicines for nausea attempt to curb it either through the nervous system, or through neutralization of the nauseating toxins in the stomach. This blend appears to work at both levels, a determination that was verified only after years of research. The primary effects of this blend are due to the Ginger root. Licorice root is added for its gastrointestinal healing properties. A minute amount of Cayenne is present for its pleasantly stimulating effect. In earlier versions of this blend, I combined the Ginger root with other carminatives, such as fennel, catnip and peppermint, all good herbs in their own right. However, none of them were as good as Ginger root; they only served to dilute the Ginger root. Licorice root and Cayenne, however, provide properties that Ginger root does not possess, and actually potentiate the activity and effectiveness of the Ginger root.

GINGER ROOT has been the subject of my intense interest, both professional and avocational, for several years. Eventually, a colleague and I published a paper on the effects of Ginger root on motion sickness (1). Compared to dimenhydrinate, the most common over-the-counter drug, Ginger root was significantly better. But that's just one kind of nausea. Briefly, here is a summary of my findings on the effects of Ginger root on various types of nausea, involving the participation of literally hundreds of people, over a period of eight years.

1. Motion Sickness. The herb worked for over 90% of the people who used it correctly. It was most effective when 2-4 capsules were ingested prior to travel. Two more capsules were ingested about every hour or so, or immediately upon feeling the least sign of upset stomach.

2. Morning Sickness. Ginger root was effective in reducing or eliminating morning sickness in just over 75% of the cases. Generally, the women who had the most success took anywhere from 3-8 capsules before getting out of bed in the morning, then stayed in bed and kept taking the herb (up to the 8-10 capsule range) until any nausea they felt upon waking was gone. Throughout the day, they took 3-5 capsules at the slightest hint of nausea, and then relaxed quietly until the nausea went away.

3. Dizziness and Vertigo. Not only did Ginger root prevent nausea, but it eliminated dizziness as well in 40-50% of the cases I observed. About half a dozen cases involved people who were unable to leave their homes, ride in a car or train for years. If they did they got hopelessly dizzy and then terribly sick. They took Ginger root to help subdue the nausea, and were amazed to have the vertigo disappear also. Compared to doses required for other conditions, very little Ginger root was required, usually 2-4 capsules periodically during the day.

4. Stomach Flu. Here's where people have needed the largest doses. Effective treatment regimens have gone like this: At the *very first* sign of nausea, or even sooner, if the patients suspected they were in line for a contagious virus, they took a "handful" (probably anywhere from 6 to 10) of capsules, and then 2-4 every half hour or hour, until they were certain the danger period had passed. The problem with *preventing illness is, without sophisticated tests, you can't prove you would have become ill anyway. But those who tried it, knew. The motto, if any, is: Catch it early and don't skimp on the dosage. Remember, 12 capsules equals only a tablespoon full, and we're dealing with a whole herb, not an extract.*

5. Other Conditions. In my observations and studies, *Ginger Root* has effectively eliminated headaches, remedied certain learning disabilities, and been as effective in eliminating diarrhea as it is in preventing nausea.

Toxicity. One could legitimately wonder what side effects are going to arise if people all across the land are ingesting large quantities of Ginger root. After performing toxicity tests in scores of rats and mice, I did not observe even slight toxic symptoms at doses 10 times those that human would normally ingest. To my knowledge, no other study exists that shows toxicity. Lethal dosage levels have been established, but are so high that the herb has been accepted as completely safe by the FDA. Out of the hundreds of human trials I have observed, no toxic effects have been manifested. I know people who use this blend on a daily basis, to treat chronic problems, without the slightest indication of a side effect. They tell me, "Take away my Ginger root only at the risk of *your* life." So I let them keep it.

OTHER NUTRIENTS

VITAMINS
(Daily requirements unless otherwise noted)
Pantothenic Acid *100-200 mg*
Vitamin B1 *25 mg*
Vitamin B2 *25 mg*
Vitamin B6 *100 mg*
cNiacinamide *100 mg*

MINERALS
Potassium
Calcium/Magnesium
PhosphorousLiver

MISCELLANEOUS

REFERENCES

1. Mowrey, D.B. & Clayson, D.E. "Motion sickness, ginger and psychophysics." **The Lancet,** March 20, 655-657, 1982.

NERVES & GLANDS

HERBS: **GOLDENSEAL** root (*Hydrastis canadensis*), **GENTIAN** root (*Gentiana lutea*), **Chamomile flowers** (*Matricaria chamomilla*), **Blue Vervain** (*Verbena hastata*), **Dandelion root** (*Taraxacum officinale*), **Yellow Dock root** (*Rumex crispus*), **Skullcap** (*Scutellaria lateriflora*), **Wood Betony** (*Stachys officinalis*), **Kelp** (*Laminaria, Macrocystis, Ascophyllum*), **Cayenne** (*Capsicum annum*), **Saw Palmetto berries** (*Serenoa repens-sabal*).

Form: Capsule, Tea

PURPOSE: Nerve and gland tonic.

Other Applications: Infections, Fevers, Anxiety, Insomnia, Inflammations, Anorexia, Indigestion.

USE: 2-4 capsules per day.

Contraindications: None.

This blend is meant to be a general dietary supplement, to be used on a daily basis, by virtually anyone engaged in the process of toning up the body's general functions, improving the overall health of the nerves and glands, or recovering from illness. The blend contains several clinically and scientifically verified tonics for the glands and nerves.

GOLDENSEAL has been called a cure-all, a panacea, and God's gift to mankind. When consumed in small quantities, on a regular basis, it is an effective neural and glandular tonic. Its active principles include potent antibiotics, vasoconstrictors and uterine tonics. Goldenseal has acquired an international reputation, occurring in over a dozen foreign pharmacopoeias. *(See also VAGINAL YEAST INFECTION, STOMACH/INTESTINAL, FEVERS & INFECTIONS, INFLUENZA, EYES, HEMORRHOIDS.)*

GENTIAN ROOT is a simple bitter. All bitters reflexively stimulate the activity of the glands, but each in its own way. Gentian is one of the best understood, acting on the whole digestive process, to stimulate appetite and increase digestion by stimulating the flow of bile. Simple dyspepsia, or severe anorexia, can be effectively treated by this herb. German scientists have been intensively studying Gentian root for decades. Their findings confirm the herb's tonic qualities (**1-2**). *(See also DIABETES, CIRCULATION, THYROID, STOMACH/INTESTINAL.)*

CHAMOMILE is one of the best-known "cure-alls." It is a bitter tonic with many proven properties, including antispasmodic (**3**), anti-inflammatory (**4**). and very good sedative properties (**5**). Other proven actions of the herb include anti-ulcer, antibacterial, and antimycotic effects. The traditional roles of a bitter, including a stimulating effect on the liver (**6**), have also been firmly established. Chamomile has other important functions, the most important of wwhich are anti-tumor or anti-cancer properties (e.g., **7**). Cultures as divergent as Western Europe, Russia, and India have all used Chamomile for very similar tonic purposes down through the centuries. *See also FEMALE TONIC)*

BLUE VERVAIN has been used in folk medicine as a diuretic for edema, as an antidiarrheic, a stimulant, emmenagogue, diaphoretic, expectorant, for chronic bronchitis, rheumatism, nervous pains, sleeplessness, tiredness and anemia. The herb has a weak parasympathetic mimicking activity, which probably accounts for most of the traditionally observed effects. It has been shown to contract smooth muscles of the uterus and gastro-intestinal tract, with very little toxicity (**8**). Vervain has also been proven to be anti-inflammatory and analgesic (pain killer) (**9**).

DANDELION ROOT is another effective bitter that has been used as a tonic and blood cleanser for hundreds of years, especially in Europe and China. All of the glands involved in any way with the digestive system respond rapidly and effectively to Dandelion. The many properties of Dandelion are covered in the following chapters: SKIN; DIABETES; BLOOD PURI/DETOX; LIVER DISORDERS

YELLOW DOCK ROOT achieves its tonic properties through the astringent purification of the blood supply to the glands. It is often used in seasonal cleanses and other blood detoxification programs. It has one of the strongest reputations for clearing up skin problems, liver and gall bladder ailments, and glandular inflammation and swelling. High in iron, Yellow Dock is an effective tonic treatment for anemia. *(See also SKIN; BLOOD PURIFICATION & DETOXIFICATION)*

SKULLCAP is a favorite herb among those who have discovered its effectiveness in treating numerous ailments. Its use as a tonic is derived from its bitter principles, although its calmative property is probably due to the presence of a volatile oil, scutellarin. Skullcap was used by several American Indian tribes and was listed in the National Formulary and U.S. Pharmacopoeia for a while.

WOOD BETONY was used in medieval England to cure "monstrous nocturnal visions, devils, despair and lunacy". Among these early peoples, Wood Betony was one of the most highly prized of herbs, for it could be used to keep the world sane and safe. Today, we believe that man's ability to deal with the pressures of everyday life are mainly functions of his physical health. We have also discovered the hypotensive properties of Wood Betony. So, today we use the herb to calm the nerves, encourage relaxing sleep, and tone up glandular functioning. *(See also PAIN; NERVOUS TENSION)*

KELP is an important general nutritive tonic. Until recent years it was eaten almost exclusively and universally by the Japanese. Cultural studies have determined what differences the Japanese intake of Kelp has made. Heading the list is a dramatically lower breast cancer rate. Also on the list are : less obesity, heart disease, respiratory disease, rheumatism and arthritis, high blood pressure, thyroid deficiency, constipation and gastro-intestinal ailments, and infectious disease. See the following chapters for details on Kelp: *(See also DIABETES; PROSTATE; FEVERS & INFECTIONS; WEIGHT LOSS; FATIGUE; BLOOD PURI/DETOX; HEART; PAIN; INFERTILITY; MENTAL ALERTNESS/SENILITY; ENVIRONMENTAL POLLUTION)*

CAYENNE has positive effects on circulation, the heart, the stomach and all other systems of the body. But it is not usually thought of as a tonic. It is generally considered a carminative and a stimulant. The stimulant property, however, is so prevalent that increased tonus of nerves and glands is a major end result of its action. *(See also FATIGUE; CIRCULATION; HIGH BLOOD PRESSURE)*

SAW PALMETTO BERRY is an old American tonic, dating at least as far back as the Maya. John Lloyd, a famous early American medicinal botanist, observed that animals fed on these berries grew sleek and fat. Many settlers fed them to their stock with the same remarkable results. Soon, medical researchers had verified the claims. Many articles were published reporting Saw Palmetto berry's effects on body weight, general health and disposition, tranquilization, appetite stimulation, and reproductive health. *(See also INFERTILITY; RESPIRATORY AILMENTS; DIABETES; FEMALE TONIC; PROSTATE; THYROID; DIGESTION)*

OTHER NUTRIENTS

VITAMINS
(Daily requirements unless otherwise noted) Vitamin B-1 25-100 mg
Vitamin B-2 *25-100 mg*
Vitamin B-6 *25-100 mg*
Vitamin C *500-1,000 mg*
Vitamin D *400 I.U.*
Vitamin E *400-600 I.U.*
Niacinamide *100 mg*
Folic acid *400 mcg*
Pantothenic Acid *100 mg*
    Calcium/Magnesium
    Phosphorus
    Zinc

REFERENCES

1. Glatzel, H. "Treatment of dyspeptic disorders with spice extracts." **Hippokrates**, 40(23), 916-919, 1969.
2. Deininger, R. "Amarum-bitter herbs. Common bitter principle remedies and their action." **Krankenplege**, 29(3), 99-100, 1975.
3. Verzarne, P.G., Szegi, J. & Marczal, G. "Effect of certain chamomile compounds." **Acta Pharmaceutica Hungarica**, 49(1), 13-20, 1979.
4. Jakovlev, V., Isacc, O., Thiemer, K. & Kunde, R. "Pharmacological investigations with compounds of chamomile. II. New investigations on the antiphlogistic effects of (-)-alpha-bisabolols and bisabolol oxides." **Planta Medica**, 35(2), 125-140, 1979.
5. Loggia, R.D., Traversa, U., Scarcia, V. & Tubaro, A. "Depressive effects of chamomilla recutita (l.) rausch, tubular flowers, on central nervous system in mice." **Pharmacological Research Communications**, 14(2), 153-162, 1982.
6. Pasechnik, I.K. "Choleretic action of matricaria officinalis." **Farmakilogiia i Toksikologiia**, 468-469, 1969.
7. Kraul, M.A. & Schmidt, F. "The growth-inhibiting effect of certain extracts from flores chamomilae and of a synthetic azulene derivative on experimental mice tumors." **Archive der Pharmazie (Weinheim)**, 290, 66-75, 1957.
8. List, P.H. & Hoerhammer, L. **Hagers Handbuch der Pharmazeutischen Praxis**. Volumes 2-5, Springer-Verlag, Berlin.
9. Sakai, S. "Pharmacological actions of verbena officinalis extracts." **Gifu Ika Daigaku Kiyo**, 11(1), 6-17, 1963.

NERVOUS TENSION

HERBS: **VALERIAN** root (*Valeriana officinalis*), **Passion Flower** (*Passiflora incarnata*), **Wood Betony** (*Stachys officinalis*), **Black Cohosh root** (*Cimicifuga racemosa*), **Skullcap** (*Scutellaria lateriflora*), **Hops** (*Humulus lupulus*), **Ginger root** (*Zingiber officinale*).

Form: Capsule.

PURPOSE: Nervine and calmative for anxiety, fear, being overworked, hysteria and other problems aggravated by emotional disturbances.

Other Applications: Insomnia, childhood hyperactivity, psychosomatic problems, restlessness.

USE: 1. 2-3 caps every four hours as needed.
2. Insomnia: 2 caps 2 hours before retiring; 2 caps upon retiring. Or use INSOMNIA blend.
3. Hyperactivity: 2 caps at breakfast and lunch.

Contraindications: None. Used alone or in conjunction with other blends and medications, this blend is completely safe.

This blend contains a group of safe herbs whose sedative properties are known throughout the world. Only in an encapsulated product such as this could they all be so easily combined. This blend can be expected to provide mild sedation and tranquilization at the recommended usage. Although some of the herbs in this blend are significant relaxants and sedatives by themselves, most of these herbs work best in combination.

VALERIAN ROOT, as well as its valepotriate constituents, are tranquilizing on the nervous system. For centuries man has used this plant to calm upset nerves, treat psychological disorders, pain and headache. The herb is a proven sedative; but it also improves coordination, and antagonizes the hypnotic effects of alcohol (**1**). It also has a marked tendency to increase concentration ability, as well as energy level (**2**). Valmane, a German drug containing pure substances from Valerian root, has been shown to suppress and regulate the autonomic nervous system in patients with control disorders, to be mildly sedative, to help regulate psychosomatic disorders, and relieve tension and restlessness (**3**). One of the more interesting studies was performed on childhood behavior disorders. One hundred twenty children exhibiting various kinds of psychosomatic disturbances and behavioral disorders such as learning disability, hyperactivity and anxiety were treated for several weeks with Valmane. During that period over 75% experienced significant progress or complete recovery (**4**). Many other studies similar to the have been performed (e.g. *5-6), but space does not permit their review here. (See also HIGH BLOOD PRESSURE; INSOMNIA)*

PASSION FLOWER was first investigated scientifically less than 100 years ago when it was found to possess an analgesic (pain-killing) property, and to prevent, without side effects, sleeplessness caused by brain inflammation (**7**). Since then, the sedative property of Passion flower has been observed in many studes (e.g., **8-9**). *(See also INSOMNIA; FEMALE TONIC)*

WOOD BETONY was used by early American eclectic physicians as a tonic, sedative, astringent and vulnerary (wound healer) (**10**). Scientific verification is minimal. In fact, experimental work of any sort is hard to find. One study, however, did demonstrate that the glycosides of Wood Betony have observable hypotensive activity (**11**). This effect would explain most of the clinically observed properties, since a substance that is hypotensive would tend to relax nervous tension as well as loosen up constrictive blood vessels that are producing headaches, etc. *(See also PAIN; NERVES & GLANDS)*

BLACK COHOSH has hypotensive and vasodilatory properties which are firmly supported by basic research (**12-13**). Such experimental verification follows hundreds of years of using Black Cohosh for exactly the purposes finally substantiated. Black Cohosh is a primary nerve and smooth muscle relaxant and works great in cases of irritated nerves and general restlessness. *(See also FEMALE TONIC; HIGH BLOOD PRESSURE; CHOLESTEROL REGULATION)*

SKULLCAP is another good tonic and nervine, effective for insomnia, excitability, restlessness and other nervous complaints. Most research on this plant has been carried out in Russia, at most of her major universities. A typical study finds that Skullcap is hypotensive or relaxing (**14**). Some major Russian medical books discuss the scientific findings in great detail. Therein, experiments are reviewed which have proven Skullcap to be a tonic, a sedative, an anti-epileptic and so on(e.g., **15-16**). *(See also INSOMNIA; NERVES & GLANDS; PAIN)*

HOPS are one of the traditional nervine, sedative type agents employed in folk medicine throughout the Western world. Hops have also been the fortunate subject of a great deal of modern scientific investigation. One recent study showed that Hops are truly sedative, as opposed to merely muscle-relaxing (**17**). They are also fast acting. A soothing, relaxing calm will be experienced within 20-40 minutes after ingesting the herb (**18**). The earliest demonstratin of sedative action in Hops was made in 1966, after other investigators had tried unsuccessfully for many years (**19**). *(See also INSOMNIA)*

GINGER ROOT is usually used as a carminative to soothe upset stomach. Its action is not fully understood, but at least one bit of research indicates that it has cholinergic action (**20**), and would therefore serve to maintain equilibrium in the nerves, glands and muscles of a body under stress. It would tend to offset the nerve-wracking effects of stress, helping to calm the system and inhibit that "pins and needles" feeling. *(See also FATIGUE; CIRCULATION; LAXATIVE; NAUSEA; STOMACH/INTESTINAL; DIGESTION; LOW BLOOD SUGAR)*

OTHER NUTRIENTS

VITAMINS
(Daily requirements unless otherwise noted)
Vitamin B-1 *25-100 mg*
Vitamin B-2 *25-100 mg*
Vitamin B-6 *25-100 mg*
Vitamin C *500-1000 mg*
Vitamin D *400 I.U.*
Vitamin E *400-600 I.U.*
Niacinamide *100 mg*
Folic acid *400 mcg*
Pantothenic Acid *100 mg*
Choline *1-2 g*

MINERALS
Calcium/Magnesium
Phosphorus
Zinc
Potassium

MISCELLANEOUS
Lecithin
Brewer's Yeast
Essential Fatty Acid
GLA

REFERENCES

1. V. Eickstedt, K.S., et.al., **Arzneimittel-Forschungen**, 19, 316, 1969; and 19, 993, 1969.
2. Schaette, R. **Dissertation Muenchen**, 1971. and Schaette, R. "Stable valerian preparations." **Ger. Offen. 2,230,626**, 10 Jan. 1974.
3. Boeters, U. "Treatment of autonomic dysregulatioin with valepotriates (Valmane)." **Muenchener Medizinische Wochenschrift**, 37, 1873-1876, 1969.
4. Klich, R. & Gladbach, B. "Childhood behavior disorders and their treatment." **Medizinishce Welt**, 26(25), 1251-1254, 1975.
5. Straube, G. "The meaning of Valerian root in therapy." **Therapie der Gegenwart**, 107, 555-562, 1968.
6. Hoenke, E. "Concerning psychic-vegetative effects of a supposed antihistaminic." **Nervenarzt**, 37, 448-453, 1953.
7. Lutomski, J. "Alkaloidy Pasiflora incarnata L." **Dissertation , Institut for Medicinal Plant Research**, Poznan, 1960.
8. Ambuehl, H. "Anatomical and chemical investigations on Passiflora coerula L. und Passiflor incarnata L." **Diss. Nr. 3830 ETH**, Zurich, 1966.
9. Lutomski, J., Malek, B., Rybacka, L. "Pharmacological investigation of the raw materials from passiflora genus. 2. pharmacochemical estimation of juices from the fruits of passiflora edulis and passiflora edulis forma flavicarpa." **Planta Medica**, 27, 112, 1975.
10. Smith, H. H. "Ethnobotany of the Potawatomi." **Bulletin of the Public Museum**, 7, 32-127, 1933.
11. Zinchenko, T.V. & Fefer, I.M. "Investigation of glycosides from betonica officinalis." **Farmatsevt. Zhurnal**, 17(3), 35-38, 1962.
12. Salerno, G.L. **Minerva otorinolaringologica**, 155, 5.
13. Genazzani, E. & Sorrentino, L. "Vascular action of acteina: active constituent of actaea racemosa L." **Nature**, 194(4828), 544-545, 1962.
14. Usow, V. **Farmakologiia i Toksikologiia**, 21(2), 31-34, 1958.
15. Meshkovsky, M.D. **Ekarstvennye Sredstva**, (Medical Preparations), Medicina Pubs, Moscow, 1967.
16. Gammerman, A.F., Yourkevitch, I.D., Eds. **Wild Medical Plants."** Bello-Russ Pubs, Academy of Science, Institute of Experimental Botanics and Microbiology, Minsk, Bello-Russia, 1965.
17. Wohlfart, R., Haensel, R. & Schmidt, H. "An investigation of sedative-hypnotic principles in Hops. Part 4." **Planta Medica**, 48, 120-123, 1983.
18. Wohlfart, R., Haensel, R. &Schmidt, H. "An investigation of sedative-hypnotic principles in Hops, Part 3." **Planta Medica**, 45, 224, 1982.
19. Berndt, G. **Deutsche Apotheker Zietung**, 106, 158, 1966.
20. Suzuki, Y., Kajiyama, K., Taguchi, K., Hagiwara, Y. & Imada, Y. "Pharmacological studies on Zingiber mioga (1) General pharmacological effects of water extracts." **Folia Pharmacologia Japonia**, 75, 669-682, 1979.

PAIN RELIEF

HERBS: **WHITE WILLOW** bark, (*Salix alba*), **Wood Betony** (*Stachys officinalis*), **Skullcap** (*Scutellaria lateriflora*), **Rosemary leaves** (*Rosmarinus officinalis*), **Raspberry leaves** (*Rubus idaeus*), **Blue Vervain** (*Verbena hastata*), & **Kelp** (*Laminaria, Macrocystis, Ascophyllum*).

Form: Capsule.

PURPOSE: To provide relief from minor pain (analgesic).

Other Applications: Headache (migraine and tension), neuralgia, neuritis, rheumatism, gout, to reduce fever, anxiety.

USE: 4-12 capsules per day, as needed (see text below).

Contraindications: None.

This blend contains the best analgesics the plant kingdom has to offer, short of habituating alkaloids like morphine. But for every ten people, there are ten kinds of pain. The treatments of pain reflect the causes of pain. Play around with the dosage if you don't get immediate results (but never take more than 12-15 capsules/day). While all the herbs in this blend contribute in their own way to the relief of pain, White willow bark has the most immediate effect.

WHITE WILLOW BARK is the original source of salicin—the forerunner of aspirin, though weaker in activity. Down through the ages, well before the discovery of salicin, White Willow bark was used to combat pain of many different sorts, including rheumatism, headache, fever, arthritis, gout, and angina. It is mentioned in ancient Egyptian, Assyrian and Greek manuscripts, and was used to combat pain and fevers by Galen, Hippocrates and Dioscorides. Many native American tribes used it for headache, fever, sore muscles, rheumatism and chills. In the middle 1700's it was used to treat malaria. Aspirin, after its discovery and development, was shown to be effective against general pain, as well as the pain of rheumatism, gout and neuralgia. Incidentally, used in the raw form, the bark yields other decomposition products of salicin that may enhance the analgesic, antipyretic, disinfectant and antiseptic properties of the product.

WOOD BETONY has had many folk uses over the past 400 years, in which a mild analgesic effect can be noted, including those of antidiarrhetic, carminative, astringent, and sedative. It has been used for heartburn, gout, nervousness, catarrh, bladder and kidney stones, asthma and fatigue. Among the eclectic physicians of the last century it was a much used medicinal plant. Significant hypotensive activity has been found in the constituents of Wood Betony (**1**), but much more research is necessary before this plant's full gamut of activity can be known. *(See also NERVOUS TENSION; NERVES & GLANDS)*

SKULLCAP has a checkered history for pain relief. Some cultures strongly recommend it for the relief of headache and related pain, while other cultures overlook this application entirely. Many physicians of the 19th Century used Skullcap with great success, to treat nervous diseases, convulsions, neuralgia, insomnia, restlessness and even tetanus. These uses have persisted till the present day, but again little scientific research has been carried out. In one study, it was found to stabilize and normalize blood pressure (**2**). This may explain why it is usually recommended for pain associated with nervous conditions. It may best be considered a minor neural sedative. *(See also INSOMNIA; NERVOUS TENSION; NERVES & GLANDS)*

ROSEMARY LEAF has been effectively used in Europe and China to treat headaches and stomach pains. A few years ago, Italian researchers demonstrated moderate analgesic activity in this herb (**3**). The oil contributes substantially to the calming and soothing of tense nerves and muscles. In China, Rosemary Leaf is used as an analgesic, smooth muscle stimulant, headache remedy, and antimalarial.

BLUE VERVAIN was shown in 1964 to have definite analgesic and antiinflammatory activity (**4**). The demonstration of these properties confirmed folk uses of the herb that dated back hundreds of years. Verbenalin, one of the active principles of Vervain, has moderate parasympathetic properties, i.e., it has a calming, restorative effect on the nervous system (**5**). *(See also NERVES & GLANDS; FEVERS & INFECTIONS(*

KELP is useful in this blend as a provider of iodine, vitamins and minerals. The prevention of painful conditions such as rheumatism and arthritis can sometimes be accomplished through nutrition. We know, for example, that an excess of acid-forming foods can precipitate painful episodes, as in the case of uric acid contribution to rheumatic pain. Acidity and lack of essential nutrients that insure the health of the nerves and their insulating sheaths can lead to inflammation and neuritis. Iodine, acting as a tranquilizer, can interrupt the physical chain that goes disease-to-pain-to-aggravation-more disease-more pain, etc.

OTHER NUTRIENTS

VITAMINS
(Daily requirements unless otherwise noted)
- Vitamin B Complex
- Vitamin B1 *25 mg*
- Vitamin B2 *25 mg*
- Vitamin B6 *25 mg*
- Vitamin E *400 I.U.*
- Pantothenic Acid *100 mg*
- Niacinamide *25 mg*

MINERALS
- Calcium/Magnesium
- Phosphorous

REFERENCES

1. Zinchenko, T.C., & Fefer, I.M. "Investigation of glcosides from Betonica officinalis." **Farmatsevt. Zhurnal**, 17(3), 35-38, 1962.
2. Usow, T. **Farmakologiia i Toksikologiia**. 21(2), 31-34, 1958.
3. Boido, A., Sparatore, F., Biniecka, M. "N-substituted derivatives of rosmaricine." **Studi Sassar., Sez 2**, 53(5-6), 383-93, 1975.
4. Sakai, S. "Pharmacological actions of verbena officinalis extracts." **Gifu Ika Daigaku Kiyo**, 11(1), 6-17, 1963.
5. Thomson, W.R. **Herbs that Heal**, Charles Scribner's Sons, New York, 1976.

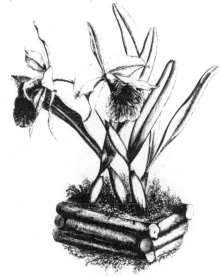

PARASITES & WORMS

HERBS: GARLIC (*Allium sativum*), BLACK WALNUT (*Juglans nigra*), Butternut bark of root (*Juglans cinera*).

Form: Capsule

PURPOSE: Parasites and worms (not intended for external application).

Other Applications: Snakebites, trauma, shock.

USE: 2 3 caps, four times per day until problem is eliminated.

Contraindications: None.

Parasitic infections arise from the intrusion of roundworms, tapeworms, protozoa and flukes into the body. They enter via the mouth or the skin. They are found in contaminated soil, vegetables, meat, water, watercress, and feces. Symptoms include colicky pains, diarrhea, anemia, cardiac insufficiency, nausea, perianal & perineal pruritis, dysentery, amebic hepatitis, weight loss, intestinal toxemia, colic and cirrhosis. There are many pharmaceutical preparations available for dealing with parasites, but the plant kingdom provides some agents that are safer to use, and just as effective. All three herbs in this blend have at one time or another been used in medical practice to kill and/or expel worms from the G.I. tract. There are many other vermifuges (parasite killers) and anthelmintics (parasite expellers) in the plant kingdom; most are caustic, toxic or simply too noxious to use. This blend was chosen for both the sureness and the mildness of its total action.

GARLIC is used by Eastern and Western cultures to kill and expel parasites and worms. Many American Indians benefited from this property of Garlic, as did the Greeks and Romans. And some of the early American physicians successfully destroyed worms with Garlic. The presence of allicin, the odoriferous principle, and allyl sulfide is responsible for this and many other beneficial properties (e.g., **1**). Roundworms, pinworms, tapeworms and hookworms all succumb to the volatile powers of Garlic (**2**). You may on occasion even find this herb in an ointment for external application against ringworm. *(See also FEVERS & INFECTIONS; HIGH BLOOD PRESSURE)*

BLACK WALNUT BARK, including the kernel and green hull have been used to expel various kinds of worms by the Asians, as well as by some American Indian tribes. External applications have been made to kill ringworm (**3**). The Chinese use it to kill tapeworm with extremely good success (**4**). There are stories going around about the ability of Black Walnut to protect people from electrocution because it contains ellagic acid. These tales may be misleading. Although only small amounts of ellagic acid are found in Black Walnut, relatively large doses were used in studies that found that it could both lower blood pressure, and, paradoxically, block the lowering of blood pressure by other agents (**5-7**). In addition, if injected intravenously, ellagic acid produced sedation and protected mice from death after a normally lethal degree of electroconvulsive shock (**8**). It is extremely doubtful that any of these effects would show up in humans ingesting whole herb material. It is more likely that the minute amount of ellagic acid in the whole herb would be metabolically neutralized long before it was absorbed by the tissues of the body. The same team found that *several* constituents of Black Walnut, including ellagic acid, juglone, several strong and weak acids, and alkaloids, had anti-cancer properties (**9**). More work in this later area could have been most fruitful, but was never pursued.

BUTTERNUT BARK OF ROOT, or White walnut, is used to expel, rather than kill, worms (vermifuge) during the normal coarse of laxative-induced cleansing. When combined with anthelmintics, Butternut bark of root provides the means to eliminate the parasitic mass from the body. These properties were known in America in the early 1800's and probably even earlier (**10**). Mode of action is not known. *(See also LAXATIVE; FEVERS & INFECTIONS)*

OTHER NUTRIENTS

VITAMINS
(Daily requirements unless otherwise noted)
Vitamin A *25,000 I.U.*
Vitamin B Complex
Vitamin B1 *25-100 mg*
Vitamin B2 *25-100 mg*
Vitamin B6 *25-100 mg*
Vitamin B12 *5 mcg*
Vitamin D *1,000 I.U.*
Pantothenic Acid *100 mg*

MINERALS
Calcium/Magnesium
Iron
Potassium

MISCELLANEOUS
GLA
Essential Fatty Acid
Cod Liver Oil
Brewer's yeast

REFERENCES

1. Yamada, Y. & Azuma, K. "Evaluation of the in vitro antifungal activity of allicin." **Antimicrobial Agents Chemotherapy**, 11, 743, 1977.
2. Rao, RR., Rao, S.S. & Venkatoraman, P.R. **Journal Scient. Ind. Res.**, 5, 31, 1946.
3. Harris, W.R. **Practice of medicine and surgery by the Canadian tribes in Champlain's time.** 27th ann. Archeol. Rep. Min. Educ., Ontario, 1915 (written in 1900).
4. Leung, A.Y. **Chinese Herbal Remedies**, Universe Books, New York, 1984.
5. Bhargava, U.C. "Pharmacology of ellagic acid from black walnut." From **Dissertation Abstracts B**, 29(1), 294-295, 1967.
6. Bhargava, U.C. & Westfall, B.A. "Antagonistic effect of ellagic acid on histamine liberators." **Proceedings of the Society of Experimental Biology and Medicine**, 131(4), 1342-1345, 1969.
7. Bhargava, U.C., & Westfall, B.A. "Mechanism of blood pressure depression by ellagic acid." **Proceedings of the Society of Experimental Biology and Medicine**, 132(2), 754-756, 1969.
8. Bhargava, U.C., Westfall, B.A. & Siehr, D.J. "Preliminary pharmacology of ellagic acid from juglans nigra (black walnut)." **Journal of Pharmaceutical Sciences**, 57(10), 1728-1732, 1968.
9. Bhargava, U.C. & Westfall, B.A. "Antitumor activity of juglans nigra (black walnut) extractives." **Journal of Pharmaceutical Sciences**, 57(10), 1674-1677, 1968.
10. Rafinesque, C.S. **Medical Flora or Manual of Medical Botany of the United States.** Vol 2., Atkinson & Alexander, Philadelphia, 1830.

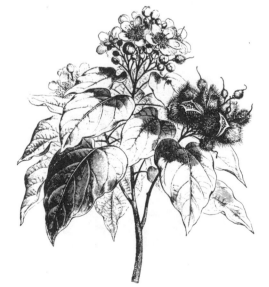

PROSTATE PROBLEMS

HERBS: **PARSLEY** (*Petroselinum sativum*), **SAW PALMETTO** berries (*Serenoa repens-sabal*), **Cornsilk** (*Stigmata maydis*), **Buchu leaves** (*Barosma crenata*), **Cayenne** (*Capsicum annum*), **Kelp** (*Laminaria, Macrocystis, Ascophyllum*), & **Pumpkin seeds** (*Curcurbita pepo*).

Form: Capsule.

PURPOSE: Prostate problems: enlarged and/or inflamed prostate.

Other Applications: Diuretic.

USE: 1. Inflamed prostate: 4-8 caps/day.
2. Enlarged prostate: 3-6 caps/day.

Contraindications: None. Exercise care when using any diuretic type preparation as they can cause serum potassium depletion if used in large amounts for an extended period of time.

This blend helps fight infected prostate (prostatitis) and enlarged prostate (hypertrophy) in at least four ways. First, it acts to stimulate urine flow when an enlarged prostate is inhibiting such flow. Second, it helps reduce inflammation and infection. Third, it helps decrease the size of the enlarged prostate. Fourth, it helps prevent these conditions. When the enlarged prostate clamps around the urethra this blend will promote urination, soothe irritated tissues reduce inflammation and pain and curb that dull aching throb.

PARSLEY is the foremost diuretic to be recommended when urination is painful and incomplete due to an enlarged prostate squeezing the urethra so tightly that urination is difficult. The presence of apiol and myristicin as well as other flavanoids in Parsley will stimulate urination and provide relief. There is much talk of overdoses of pure apiol being harmful to the kidneys and liver. One need not fear poisoning from the plant itself (**1**). Parsley works best in blends with other herbs, such as Buchu and Cornsilk. *(See also DIABETES; DIURETIC; BONE-FLESH-CARTILAGE)*

SAW PALMETTO BERRY acts directly on the enlarged prostate to reduce inflammation, pain and throb (**5**). It also increases the bladder's ability to contract and expel its contents (**6**). Credit for the discovery of these principles goes to the early American eclectic physicians who so effectively transformed native American flora into a medicinal storehouse. *(See also INFERTILITY; RESPIRATORY AILMENTS; DIABETES; FEMALE PROBLEMS; NERVES & GLANDS; THYROID; DIGESTION)*

CORNSILK is a diuretic and acts much like parsley. It is contained in several over-the-counter type diuretic products in Europe and America (where it use to be an officially recognized medicinal agent), and is popular in China also. Most herbalists around the world agree that Cornsilk directly reduces painful symptoms and swelling due to several inflammatory conditions, including cystitis, pyelitis, oligouria, hepatitis, and all edematous conditions. *(See also DIURETIC)*

BUCHU LEAF is provided as a urinary disinfectant, one of the important secondary considerations when treating prostate problems. By themselves, Buchu leaves are seldom used for acute prostate problems, but they lend just the right antiseptic property to preparations used for acute as well as chronic prostate problems. South Buchu works because

its volatile oil stimulates urination and is excreted virtually unchanged by the kidneys, rendering the urine slightly antiseptic (**9**). Proprietary drugs are available in South Africa and the United States that still employ Buchu leaves as a urinary antiseptic DIURETIC; VAGINAL YEAST INFECTION

CAYENNE is included in this blend once again as a mild systemic stimulant to insure the diffusion of the active principles of other herbs throughout the body via the vascular system.

KELP has been used for scores of years by Asian peoples to treat disorders of the genital-urinary tract, including kidney, bladder, prostate and uterine problems. Clinical documentation is available to show that Kelp ingestion on a daily basis gradually reduces the prostate in older men to the point that urination becomes painless, even though it is not certain how that occurs (**11**). *(See also THYROID; CIRCULATION; ENVIRONMENTAL POLLUTION; FEVERS & INFECTIONS; WEIGHT LOSS; FATIGUE; BLOOD PURIFICATION/DETOXIFICATION; HEART; INFERTILITY; PAIN; MENTAL ALERTNESS/SENILITY; DIABETES)*

PUMPKIN SEED has a reputation of being a non-irritating diuretic. This property makes the seed especially well suited to treat the enlarged prostate. Native American Indians used it successfully for this purpose long before the settlers adopted it for their own purposes (**15**). Today, it is universally accepted for this specific purpose (though its main use continues to be as an anthelmintic).

OTHER NUTRIENTS

VITAMINS
(Daily requirements unless otherwise noted)
Vitamin A *25,000 I.U.*
Vitamin B-1 *25-100 mg*
Vitamin B-2 *25-100 mg*
Vitamin B-6 *25-100 mg*
Vitamin C *1,000-5,000 mg*
Vitamin E *600 I.U.*

MINERALS
Zinc

REFERENCES

1. List, P.H. & Hoerhammer, L. **Hagers Handbuch der Pharmazeutischen Praxis.** Volumes 2-5, Springer-Verlag, Berlin.
2. Felter, H. W. **The Eclectic Materia Medica, Pharmacology and Therapeutics.** Eclectic Medical Publications, Portland, Oregon, 1983 (first published 1922).
3. Ellingwood, F. **American Materia Medica, Therapeutics and Pharmacognosy.** Eclectic Medical Publications, Portland, Oregon, 1983.
4. Tyler, V.E., Brady, L.R. & Robbers, J.E. **Pharmacognosy**, 7th ed., Lea & Febiger, Philadelphia, 1976.
5. Personal communication from Dr. H. Tamamoto, Tokyo, Japan, 1983.6. Vogel, V.J. *American Indian Medicine.* Ballantine Books, New York, 1970.

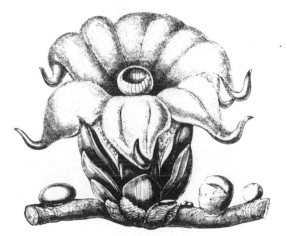

RESPIRATORY AILMENTS

HERBS: PLEURISY ROOT (*Asclepias tuberosa*), **Wild Cherry bark** (*Prunus virginiana*), **Slippery Elm bark** (*Ulmus fulva*), **Plantain** (*Plantago ovata*), **Mullein leaves** (*Verbascum thapsus*), **Chickweed** (*Stellaria media*), **Horehound** (*Marrubium vulgare*), **Licorice root** (*Glycyrrhiza glabra*), **Kelp** (*Laminaria, Macrocystes, Ascophyllum*), **Cayenne** (*Capsicum annuum*), & **Saw Palmetto** (*Serenoa serrulata*).

Form: Capsule, Gargle, Tea, Mouthwash

PURPOSE: To relieve the distress of respiratory ailments, such as pneumonia, asthma, bronchitis, croup, tuberculosis, colds, flu, hayfever, emphysema (acts to soothe, tone, and relieve irritation).

Other Applications: Allergies, fevers, colitis.

USE: 1. To relieve general respiratory distress: 4-6 caps/day.
2. As a tea: 2-4 caps/cup. 3. As a gargle: 2 caps/cup.

Contraindications: None. Due to mild diuretic action, consider potassium supplementation.

Although this blend is meant primarily as a treatment for the symptoms, some of the herbs have been shown to remedy and/or prevent some forms of respiratory disease itself. Virtually every herb in this blend has been shown to help relieve distress due to cough, or infection or inflammation. Simply swallowing the capsules is perhaps the least effective method of using this blend. Teas and gargles are the best methods. A bit of honey, saturated with the contents of one or two capsules is also recommended.

PLEURISY ROOT, is a much used treatment for colds, flu, bronchitis, tuberculosis, pleurisy, and so on (**1**). In America, it was the primary expectorant for several decades, said to possess "...an almost specific quality of acting on the organs of respiration, powerfully promoting...expectoration," (**2**). This enthusiasm is shared by the majority of naturopathic physicians.

WILD CHERRY BARK's use for reducing the symptoms of respiratory distress is without equal in the herb kingdom. Its widespread inclusion in over-the-counter cough medications testifies to its acceptance by the pharmaceutical and medical industries (many such preparations, however, on the mistaken assumption that the herb is just for taste, only use cherry flavoring). The real thing, the actual bark, is much more effective than most cough drop or throat lozenge-type preparations. *(See also HAYFEVER & ALLERGIES)*

SLIPPERY ELM BARK, due to its high and peculiar mucilage content, is remarkably effective, both internally and externally, against sore and inflamed mucous membranes, and is one of the best agents for combating coughs. The American Indians obtained more mileage from this herb than practically any other medication, using it variously to ease childbirth and reduce the pain of labor, for toothaches, dysentery, diarrhea, leprosy, ulcers, rheumatism, eye lotions, and all forms of external sores and wounds (**3**). *(See also BONE-FLESH-CARTILAGE; HEMORRHOIDS/ASTRINGENT)*

PLANTAIN, one of the most underrated of all herbs, is included on the basis of its similarities to the other mucilaginous herbs in this blend, and on the strength of modern research. For example, scientists recently treated a number of cases of chronic bronchitis with Plantain and found that the herb provided very good symptomatic relief of pain, coughing, wheezing and irritation (**4**). *(See also BONE-FLESH-CARTILAGE; VAGINAL YEAST INFECTION; WEIGHT LOSS; CHOLESTEROL REGULATION)*

MULLEIN LEAF is used in India for upper respiratory problems (**5**). In addition to the soothing effect imparted by the mucilage, Mullein possesses good antibiotic properties (**6**). During the Civil War, the Confederates relied on Mullein for treatment of respiratory problems whenever their medical supplies ran out. Several different and unrelated Indian tribes used Mullein for similar purposes (**3**).

CHICKWEED was another plant well-liked by the American Indians for the relief it gave for such respiratory problems as bronchitis, whooping cough, colds, sore throat and flu (**7**). It achieved near panacea status in some. In European folklore, the herb was used for very similar purposes, plus tuberculosis. Modern research on Chickweed, though scanty, has at least demonstrated the presence of antibiotic properties which are effective against certain respiratory pathogens (**1**).

HOREHOUND's popularity as a cough remedy can hardly be disputed. Not so well known is the fact that Horehound and/or its derivatives are used in virtually thousands of bronchial medications around the world. Its activity is no doubt due to a high content of volatile oil. This oil has vasodilatory, as well as expectorant properties (**8**). *(See also HAYFEVER & ALLERGIES)*

LICORICE ROOT has been the subject of numerous scientific studies involving anti-inflammatory and antitussive properties. A typical study shows that it curbs inflammations throughout the body, including the lungs and throat (**9-11**). Licorice root derivatives have been shown to be as effective as codeine in terms of suppressing coughs (**11**). Sugars, glycosides and other constituents with adrenocortical-like activity are probably responsible for its effectiveness.

SAW PALMETTO BERRY also contains anti-inflammatory principles, as well as being a strong expectorant. Its primary purpose in this blend is to remove catarrh from the mucous membranes. Saw Palmetto is best known for its effects on sexual function. *(See also INFERTILITY; DIABETES; FEMALE TONIC; PROSTATE; NERVES & GLANDS; THYROID; DIGESTION)*

KELP and **CAYENNE** provide nutritive support and stimulate circulation, thereby increasing the oxygen exchange capacity of the lungs. The nature of Cayenne is to break up mucous, promoting the expectorant nature of other herbs in the blend.

OTHER NUTRIENTS

VITAMINS
(Daily requirements unless otherwise noted)
Vitamin A 25,000 I.U.
Vitamin B Complex
Vitamin B1 25-50 mg
Vitamin B2 25-50 mg
Vitamin B6 25-100 mg
Vitamin B12 10 mcg
Vitamin C 1,000-3,000 mg
Vitamin D 600-2,000 I.U.
Vitamin E 400-800 I.U.
Choline 1,000 mg
Inositol 1,000 mg
Pantothenic Acid 150-200 mg
Niacinamide 50 mg

MINERALS
Manganese
Calcium/Magnesium
Phosphorous
Potassium
Sodium

MISCELLANEOUS
Bee Pollen
HCl
Liver
Lecithin
Yogurt

REFERENCES

1. Fitzpatrick, F.K. "Plant substances active against mycobacterium tuberculosis." **Antibiotics and Chemotherapy**, 4(5), 528-536, 1954.
2. Millspaugh, C.F. **American Medicinal Plants**. Dover Publications, Inc. New York, 1974 (originally published 1892), 540-541.
3. Vogel, V.J. *American Indian Medicine*. Ballantine Books, New York, 1970.
4. Matev, M., Angelova, I., Koichev, A., Leseva, M. & Stefanov, G. "Clinical trial of a Plantago major preparation in the treatment of chronic bronchitis." **Vutreshni Bolesti (Sofia)**, 21(2), 133-137, 1982.
5. Chopra, R.N., Nayar, S.L. & Chopra, I.C. **Glossary of Indian Medicinal Plants**. Council of Scientific & Industrial Research, New Delhi, India, 1956.
6. Fitzpatrick, F.K. "Plant substances active against mycobacterium tuberculosis." **Antibiotics and Chemotherapy**, 4(5), 528-536, 1954.
7. Scully, V. **A Treasury of American Indian Herbs**. Bonanza Books, New York, 1960, 212-213.
8. Karryev, M.O., Bairyev, C.B. & Ataeva, A.S. "Some therapeutic properties and phytochemistry of common horehound." Izvestiia Akademii Nauk Turkm. SSSR, Seriia Biologicheskaia,, 3, 86-88, (1976).
9. Nasyrov, K.M. & Lazareva, D.N. "Anti-inflammatory activity of glycyrrhizic acid derivatives." **Farmakologiia i Toksikologiia** 1980, 43(4), 399-404.
10. Lutomski, J. "Chemistry and therapeutic use of licorice (Glycyrrhiza glabra L.)" **Pharmazie in Unserer Zeit**, 1983, 1(8339), 1442.
11. Anderson, D.M. & Smith, W.G., "The antitussive activity of glycyrrhetinic acid and its derivatives." **Journal of Pharmacy and Pharmacology**. 13, 1961, 396-404.

SKIN DISORDERS

HERBS: **CHAPARRAL** (*Larrea divaricata*), **DANDELION** root (*Taraxacum officinale*), **Burdock root** (*Arctium lappa*), **Licorice root** (*Glycyrrhiza glabra*), **Echinacea** (*Echinacea purpurea*), **Yellow Dock root** (*Rumex crispus*), **Kelp** (*Laminaria, Macrocystes, Ascophyllum*), & **Cayenne** (*Capsicum annuum*).

Form: Capsule, Poultice, Compress

PURPOSE: For skin disorders; Rash; Itch; Psoriasis; General cleansing; Eczema; Acne Vulgaris; Dry and scaly skin.

Other Applications: Almost any skin disease.

USE: 1. General Cleansing: 2-3 caps, 3-4 times per day.
2. For serious skin conditions: 6-8 caps/day, supplemented by additional Chaparral, Dandelion and Echinacea.
3. An excellent blood purification program is 3-4 capsules per day of this blend, and the same amount of the ARTHRITIS and BLOOD PURIFICATION/DETOXIFICATION blends.
4. With the BONE-FLESH-CARTILAGE Blend: 3 caps/day.

Contraindications: None. Chaparral, though often called creosote bush, contains **no** creosote.

This blend attacks external skin disorders from within, purifying the blood, carrying away waste, reinforcing the blood's ability to ward off infectious agents. Several of the herbs in this blend constituted the fundamental treatment for diseases like typhoid, diptheria, cholera, syphilis and malignant skin conditions during the last century. Widespread use resulted in the documentation of a number of other uses. The assumption was that "bad blood", blood poisoning, and tissue alteration due to infectious diseases are the culprits in many of man's problems. Purify the blood, and you've eliminated much of the problem. There is considerable evidence that other cultures developed the same uses for these herbs. Enough scientific evidence exists to justify the blend's place in modern man's medicine cabinet.

CHAPARRAL caused quite a stir in the early '70's, as it appeared that its anti-cancer properties were at last becoming scientifically proven (**1**). Animal studies strongly sugggest that Chaparral or its main constituent, NDGA (nordihydroguaiaretic acid), is toxic against cancer cells (not normal cells). The herb's effectiveness against other forms of skin diseases may be attributed to its anti-microbial properties (**2**), its ability to increase ascorbic acid levels in the adrenals (**3**), its tonic quality, or to some other, as yet undiscovered mechanism. *(See also DETOXIFY/NURTURE. ARTHRITIS; BONE-FLESH-CARTILAGE)*

DANDELION ROOT seems to have some potential for fighting cancer (**5**). The Chinese use Dandelion to treat infections, pneumonia, liver disease and cancer of the breast (**5**). The plant stimulates liver activity, thereby encouraging the elimination of toxins in the blood. It stimulates the flow of bile and the excretion of urea. *(See also LIVER DISORDERS; DIABETES; BLOOD PURI/DETOX; NERVES & GLANDS)*

BURDOCK ROOT is your all around blood purifier, its action being simple but profound. Documented effects include treatment of scurvy, venereal eruptions, leprosy, and other cankerous skin conditions (**6**). In addition to its alterative (blood building) property, it is strongly diuretic and diaphoretic. Priddy Meeks, an early American herbalist is credited with removing "a bunch" growing on the upper lip of a young girl, with a treatment consisting of equal parts of Burdock and two other herbs in this blend, Dandelion and Yellow Dock. *(See also BLOOD PURI/DETOX; DETOXIFY/NURTURE; BONE-FLESH-CARTILAGE)*

LICORICE ROOT has been firmly established by modern research as an effective skin and tissue treatment, beginning with ulcers, and extending to cancer (**8**). Topical preparations based on Licorice Root derivatives have been shown to be effective against a wide variety of skin problems, including eczematous dermatoses, contact dermatitis, anal piles, inflammatory eye conditions, pruritis, all manner of itchy inflammatory conditions, neurodermatitis, atopic eczema, lichen simplex, and infantile eczema (e.g., **9-10,**). Combined with neomycin, these preparations have cured impetigo. Topical preparations of Licorice root derivatives worked best on chronic conditions. Overall, their activity compares favorably with hydrocortisone (**11**). *(See also ARTHRITIS; RESPIRATORY AILMENTS; FEMALE TONIC; CIRCULATION; FATIGUE; BLOOD PURIFICATION/DETOXIFICATION; WEIGHT LOSS; THYROID; ENVIRONMENTAL POLLUTION; FEVERS & INFECTIONS; WHOLE BODY; MENTAL ALERTNESS/SENILITY; DETOXIFY/NURTURE)*

ECHINACEA alone accounts for hundreds of cases of reportedly cured boils, gangrene, ulcerations, animal, reptile and insect bites, abscesses and so on. Perhaps no other herb was loved and used more than this one by early American eclectic physicians. Laboratory studies show that the herb increases the ability of white blood cells to surround and destroy bacterial and viral invaders in the blood (**7**). It stimulates the lymphatic system to clean up waste material and toxins, and it has definite antimicrobial activity (**12**). *(See also BLOOD PURIFICATION/DETOXIFICATION; FEVERS & INFECTIONS)*

YELLOW DOCK ROOT is a good alterative, especially in its ability to help the body overcome chronic skin disorders like eczema, ringworm and related diseases, leprosy, psoriasis, and even cancer (**13**). As with other herbs in this blend, Yellow Dock possesses some antibiotic properties (**14**). *(See also BLOOD PURIFICATION/DETOXIFICATION; NERVES & GLANDS)*

KELP & CAYENNE are present in this blend for their stimulant and anti-infectious properties. They also supply nutritional support required for proper tissue repair.

OTHER NUTRIENTS

VITAMINS
(Daily requirements unless otherwise noted)
Vitamin A 25,000-30,000 I.U.
Vitamin B1 25-50 mg
Vitamin B2 25-50 mg
Vitamin B6 25-100 mg
Vitamin B Complex
Vitamin C 1,000-3,000 mg
Vitamin D 1,000 I.U.
Vitamin E 600-1,600 I.U.
Niacinamide 100 mg
Pantothenic Acid 200-300 mg
PABA up to 1,000 mg
Biotin 150 mg
Choline 1,000
Inositol 1,000
Folic Acid up to 5 mg

MINERALS
Zinc
Calcium/Magnesium
Potassium

MISCELLANEOUS
Essential Fatty Acids
HCl
Lecithin
Brewer's Yeast

REFERENCES

1. Smart, C.R., Hogle, H.H., Robins, R.K., Broom, A.D., & Bartholomew, D. "An interesting observation on nordihydroguaiaretic acid (NSC-4291; NDGA) and a patient with malignant melanoma—a preliminary report." **Cancer Chemotherapy Reports**, Part 1, 53, 147-151, 1969.
2. Kaufman, H.P. & Ahmad, A.K.S., **Fette, Seifen, und Anstrichmittel.**, 68, 837, 1967.
3. Sporn, A. & Schobesch, O. "Toxicity of nordihydroguaiaretic acid." **Igiena** (Bucharest), 15(12), 725-726, 1966.
4. Baba, K., Abe, S., Mizuno, D. "Antitumor activity of hot water extract of dandelion, Taraxacum officinale—correlation between antitumor activity and timing of administration." **Yakugaku Zasshi**, 101(6), 538-543, 1981.
5. **Martindale: The Extra Pharmacopoeia.** 1977. The Pharmaceutical Press. London.
6. Ellingwood, F. **American Materia Medica, Therapeutics and Pharmacognosy.** Eclectic Medical Publications, Portland, Oregon, 1983.
7. Scully, V. **A Treasury of American Indian Herbs.** Bonanza Books, New York, 1960.
8. Shvarev, I.F., Konovalova, N.K. & Putilova, G.I. "Effect of triterpenoid compounds from glycyrrhiza glabra on experimental tumors." **Voprosy Izuch. Ispol'z. Solodki SSSR. Akad. Nauk SSSR.** 167-170, 1966.
9. Adamson, A.C. & Tillman, W.G. "Hydrocortisone." **British Medical Journal**, 2, 1501, 1955.
10. Chakravorti, S. "Glycyrrhetinic acid." **British Medical Journal**, 1, 161-162, 1957.
11. Colin-Jones, E. & Somers, G.F. "Glycyrrhetinic acid, a non-steroidal anti-inflammatory agent in dermatology." **Presse Medicales** (Paris), 238, 206, 1957.
12. Samochowiez, E., Urbanska, L., Manka, W. & Stolarska, E. "Evaluation of the effect of Calendula officinalis and Echinacea augustifolia extracts on Trichomonus vaginalis in vitro." **Wiadomosci Parazytologiczne**, 25(1), 77-81, 1979.
13. Gessner, O. **Die Gift.—Arzneipflanzen von Mitteleuropa.** Heidelburg, Germany, 1931.
14. Nishikawa, H. "Screening tests for antibiotic action of plant extracts." **Japanese Journal of Experimental Medicine**, 20(3), 337-349, 1949.

STOMACH/INTESTINAL

HERBS: GOLDENSEAL root (*Hydrastis canadensis*), LICORICE root (*Glycyrrhiza glabra*), **Gentian root** (*Gentiana lutea*), **Papaya leaf** (*Carica papaya*), **Myrrh gum**, (*Commiphora myrrha*), **Irish Moss** (*Chondrus crispus*), **Fenugreek seeds** (*Trigonella foenum-graecum*), & **Ginger root** (*Zingiber officinale*).

Form: Capsule, Tea

PURPOSE: To soothe and heal gastrointestinal tract disorders, such as: Upset stomach; Gas; Heartburn; Ulcers.

Other Applications: Inflammations, Diarrhea, Giardiasis.

USE:
1. Gas, Upset Stomach: 2-4 caps as needed.
2. Chronic Heartburn: 2 caps after each meal.
3. Ulcers: 2 caps before each meal.
4. Other Applications: 2-3 caps as needed.
5. Digestion: 2 caps with meals; 2 caps of DIGESTION blend.
6. Inflammatory diseases: 2 caps with each meal.

Contraindications: Pregnant women should use NAUSEA blend.

Note: Ingest capsules with 1/2 glass of water.

This is a multi-purpose blend designed to prevent and remedy several more or less related problems of the stomach and intestinal tract. It is also a specific remedy for all kinds of ulcers, and should provide a good treatment without side effects.

GOLDENSEAL ROOT, in the opinion of many experts, can, all by itself, effectively treat indigestion, nausea, gas and heartburn. Goldenseal stimulates bile production and secretion (**1**), destroys noxious bacteria in the G.I. tract (**2**), and effectively ameliorates gastroenteritis (**3**), and diarrhea (**4**). Of concern to health officials is the increasing threat to drinking water of contamination by giardia, a pathogen that causes severe G.I. distress, with sometimes lethal consequences. Berberine is one of the very few agents that have been found to specifically remedy this ailment (**5**). *(See also INFLUENZA; VAGINAL YEAST INFECTION; NERVES & GLANDS; EYES; FEVERS & INFECTIONS; HEMORRHOIDS)*

LICORICE ROOT promotes the healing of peptic, gastric and duodenal ulcers. The primary constituent, glycyrrhetinic acid (GLA), also known as carbenoxolone sodium (CS), has become perhaps the most popular treatment world-wide for treating ulcers. CS has proved itself to be the 1 drug of choice (**6**). But it is very important to understand that Licorice root, from which 97% of the supposed active principle, GLA, has been removed, is still capable of healing ulcers, and without side effects (**7-8**). Unfortunately, whole Licorice, which must therefore possess at least two anti-ulcer principles, has not been experimentally studied at all. *(See also INFERTILITY; ARTHRITIS; RESPIRATORY AILMENTS; SKIN; FEMALE TONIC; BLOOD PURI/DETOX; CIRCULATION; FATIGUE; WEIGHT LOSS; ENVIRONMENTAL POLLUTION; FEVERS & INFECTIONS; THYROID; WHOLE BODY; DETOXIFY/NURTURE; MENTAL ALERTNESS/SENILITY)*

GENTIAN ROOT, a potent bitter, is a very good aid to digestion. This herb, in conjunction with Ginger root and lesser amounts of Wormwood and Cayenne, is effective in curing indigestion and heartburn (**9**). Gentian root stimulates the gall bladder and pancreas (**10**), causes strong stimulation of the appetite, increases saliva and digestive juice secretion, and accelerates the emptying of the stomach (**11-12**). *(See also CIRCULATION; NERVES & GLANDS; THYROID; DIGESTION)*

PAPAYA LEAF is known primarily for its digestive properties. However, it also has an anti-ulcer action. Recently, a Taiwanese research team found that animals pretreated with Papaya were significantly more resistant to stress-induced ulcers than untreated animals (**13**). The herb's tendencies to coagulate blood and to reduce acid secretion could account for these effects. *(See also DIGESTION; MENSTRUATION)*

MYRRH GUM is a disinfectant, astringent and deodorant for air passages and the urinary tract. It acts directly and rapidly on the peptic glands to increase activity, in this way increasing digestion. In cases of dyspepsia accompanied by excess mucous formation, Myrrh is highly recommended by herbalists. *(See also FEVERS & INFECTIONS; VAGINAL YEAST INFECTION)*

IRISH MOSS contains an abundance of mucilaginous essence that soothes inflamed and ulcerated surfaces. Irish Moss reduces gastric secretions and high blood pressure, and alleviates peptic and duodenal ulcers (**14**). Kelp, another marine plant, has been used for decades to effectively treat ulcers. Irish Moss also possesses anticoagulant, hypotensive and immunosuppressive properties.

FENUGREEK SEED stimulates general pancreatic secretion which should improve digestion (**15**). The mucilaginous nature of Fenugreek would act in a like fashion to Irish Moss in relieving the pain and irritation of ulcers.

Measurable improvement in general health, an increase in body weight, better protein utilization, inhibition of phosphorous secretion, and notable increases in red blood cell count can be expected through ingestion of the seeds. *(See also CHOLESTEROL REGULATION; FEMALE TONIC)*

GINGER ROOT has carminative or very soothing and mildly stimulating effects on the stomach. Use it for almost every kind of stomach discomfort, from nausea to indigestion, from simple stomachache to ulcers. Ginger root increases the flow and amylase concentration of saliva, activates peristalsis, and increases tonus of the intestinal muscles (**16**). A combination of Ginger root and Gentian root (with some Cayenne and Wormwood) is very effective in remedying indigestion and heartburn (**9**). Ginger root contains a proteolytic enzyme, zingibain, that is more effective than papain (from Papaya) or ficin. Ginger root is more effective than Dramamine in preventing motion sickness (**17**). Finally, Ginger root has been clinically proven to decrease significantly, nausea and diarrhea associated with the common three-day, or 24-hour type flus (**18**). *(See also DIGESTION; NAUSEA; LOW BLOOD SUGAR; LAXATIVE; CIRCULATION; NERVOUS TENSION; FATIGUE)*

OTHER NUTRIENTS

VITAMINS
(Daily requirements unless otherwise noted)

Vitamin A *25,000 I.U.*	Vitamin E *400 I.U.*
Vitamin B1 *25-100 mg*	Niacinamide *100 mg*
Vitamin B2 *25-100 mg*	Folic Acid *400 mcg*
Vitamin B6 *25-100 mg*	Pantothenic Acid *100-200 mg*
Vitamin C *500-1000 mg*	Inositol
Vitamin D *4,000 I.U.*	Bioflavanoids

MINERALS
Calcium/Magnesium
Potassium

MISCELLANEOUS
Lecithin
Yogurt/Acidophilus
Digestive Enzymes
Brewer's Yeast
GLA

REFERENCES

1. Kulkarni, S.K., Dandiya, P.C., Varandani, N.L. "Pharmacological investigations of berberine sulphate." **Japanese Journal of Pharmacology**, 22, 11-16, 1972.
2. Subbaiah, T.V. & Amin, A.H. "Effect of berberine sulphate on entamoeba histolytica." **Nature**, 215, 527-528, 1967.
3. Kamat, S.A. **Journal of the Association of Physicians of India**, 15, 525, 1967.
4. sharda, D.C. "Berberine in the treatment of diarrhea of infancy and childhood." **Journal of the Indian Medical Association**, 54(1), 22-24, 1970.
5. Gupte, S. "Use of berberine in the treatment of giardiasis." **American Journal of Diseases of Childhood**, 129, 866, 1975.
6. Sircus, W. "Progress report on carbenoxolone sodium." **Gut**, 13, 816-824, 1972.
7. Turpie, A.G.G., Runcie, J. & Thompson, T.J. "Clinical trial of deglycyrrhizinized liquorice in gastric ulcer." **Gut**, 10, 299-302, 1969.
8. Anderson, S., Brany, F., Caboda, J.L.F. & Mizuno, T. "Protective action of deglycyrrhizinated licorice on the occurrence of stomach ulcers in pylorus-ligated rats." **Scandanavian Journal of Gastroenterology**, 6, 683-686, 1971.
9. Glatzel, H. "Treatment of dyspeptic disorders with spice extracts." **Hippokrates**, 40(23), 916-919, 1969.
10. Deininger, R. "Amarum-bitter herbs: common bitter principle remedies and their action." **Krankenpflege**, 29(3), 99-100, 1975.
11. Glatzel, H. & Hackenberg, K. "Roentgenological studies of the effect of bitters on digestive organs." **Planta Medica**, 15(3), 223-232, 1967.
12. Yamamoto, A. in **Enzymes in Food Processing**, 2nd Ed., G. Reed, Ed., Academic Press, New York, 1975, p. 123.
13. Chen, C., Chen, S., Chow, S. & Han, P.W. "Protective effects of carica papaya Linn on the exogenous gastric ulcer in rats." **American Journal of Chinese Medicine**, 9(3), 205-212, 1981.
14. Leung, A.Y. **Encyclopedia of Common Natural Ingredients.** New York, 1980.
15. Ribes, G., Sauvaire, Y., Baccou, J.C., Valette, G., Chenon, D., Trimble, E.R. & Mariani, M.M.L. "Effects of fenugreek seeds on endocrine pancreatic secretions in dogs." **Annals of Nutrition and Metabolism**, 28, 37-43, 1984.
16. Glatzel, H. **Deutsche Apotheker Zeitung**, 110, 5, 1970.
17. Mowrey, D.B. & Clayson, D.E. "Motion Sickness, ginger, and psychophysics." **Lancet**, 1(8273), 655-657, 1982.
18. Mowrey, D.B. "The effects of ginger root on the symptoms of the common flu." Paper presented at the Rocky Mountain Psychological Association, May, 1978.

THYROID

HERBS: KELP (*Laminaria, Macrocystis, Ascophyllum*), **Gentian root** (*Gentiana lutea*), **Saw Palmetto berries** (*Serenoa repens-sabal*), **Cayenne** (*Capsicum annum*), & **Irish Moss** (*Chondrus crispus*).

Form: Capsule.

PURPOSE: A gentle tonic to heal, strengthen and maintain the Thyroid gland.

Other Applications: For the adrenal, pineal, pituitary, lymph and other glands.

USE: 1. Thyroid tonic: 2-6 caps/day as needed or desired.
2. During dieting: 1-2 caps/day.
3. For added thyroid help while using the WHOLE BODY TONIC: 1-2 caps/day.
4. With the SKIN DISORDERS blend: 2-3 caps/per day.

Contraindications: None.

An active, healthy thyroid produces hormones that are vital in maintaining normal growth and metabolism. Too much thyroid activity produces nervousness, heart palpitations and insomnia. Too little activity produces drowsiness, fatigue, impaired mental functioning, atherosclerosis, irritability, and lethargy. Severe inactivity produces obesity and coarsened features. An enlarged thyroid (usually with hyperthyroidism) is called goiter. The main thyroid hormones stimulate the activity of organs, tissues and cells, control skeletal growth and sexual development, influence the texture of skin and luster of hair, and are responsible for a person's energy or lack of it. Quite a responsibility for one gland. It is also the main repository of iodine in the body, and requires dietary iodine for proper development and functioning.

KELP, in supplying the thyroid with all the iodine it needs, increases the chances that this gland will not develop goiter, helps regulate the texture of the skin, and helps prevent dull hair. Iodine is essential for the proper regulation of energy through its effect on metabolism, i.e., by helping the body burn off excess fat (it may therefore prevent atherosclerosis that is due to disturbances in fat metabolism) (**1**). Kelp not only absorbs iodine from seawater but sponges up an enormous supply of essential nutrients, and delivers them to the thyroid gland and the rest of the body (**2**). Among the Japanese, who consume up to 25% of their diet in Kelp, thyroid disease is practically unknown, but among the Japanese who are becoming more Westernized, thyroid disease is on the rise (**4**). *(See also FEVERS & INFECTIONS; WEIGHT LOSS; FATIGUE; HEART; BLOOD PURIFICATION/DETOXIFICATION; INFERTILITY; PAIN; MENTAL ALERTNESS/SENILITY; CIRCULATION; DIABETES; PROSTATE)*

GENTIAN ROOT provides bitter principles that been known to normalize the functioning of the thyroid, probably through an indirect means. More directly, the herb stimulates the powers and organs of appetite, digestion, and assimilation. These principles are fully explained under STOMACH/INTESTINAL. *(See also DIABETES; NERVES & GLANDS; CIRCULATION)*

SAW PALMETTO BERRY assist the thyroid in regulating sexual development and in normalizing the activity of those glands and organs. The reputation of this herb is beginning to become known internationally, but research interest in other countries has not yet encompassed it. Clinical evidence, of which there is an abundance, from physicians in the modern United States is positive and enthusiastic. However, good controlled studies are presently lacking. *(See also INFERTILITY; RESPIRATORY AILMENTS; DIABETES; FEMALE TONIC; PROSTATE; NERVES & GLANDS; DIGESTION)*

CAYENNE operates by distributing nutrients, catalyzing reactions, stimulating glandular activity, and providing its own important vitamins and minerals.

IRISH MOSS, a close relative of Kelp, supplies its own quantities of iodine, trace elements and tissue salts.

OTHER NUTRIENTS

VITAMINS
(Daily requirements unless otherwise noted)
Vitamin A *25,000 I.U.*
Vitamin C *3,000-5,000 mg*
Vitamin B Complex
Vitamin E *400 I.U.*
Vitamin D *1,000 I.U.*
Pantothenic Acid *200 mg*

MINERALS
Iodine
Calcium/magnesium
Phosphorous
Potassium
Iron

MISCELLANEOUS
Water

REFERENCES

1. Guyton, A.C. **A Textbook of Medical Physiology,** 4th Ed., W.B.Saunders Co., Philadelphia, 1971.
2. Johnston, H.W. "Composition of edible seaweeds." in **Proceedings of the Seventh International Seaweed Syposium,** Wiley & Sons, New York, 1972, pp. 429-435.
3. Kagawa, Y. "Impact of westernization on the Japanese. Changes in physique, cancer, longevity and centenarians." **Preventative Medicine,** 205-217, 1978.

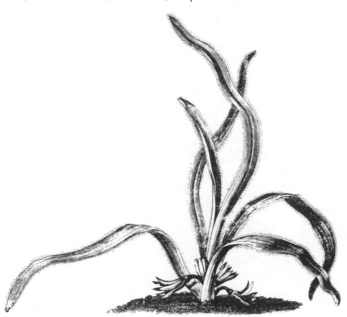

VAGINAL YEAST INFECTION

HERBS: **GOLDENSEAL** root (*Hydrastis canadensis*), **BUCHU** leaves (*Barosma crenata*), **Witch Hazel leaves** (*Hamamelis virginiana*), **Plantain** (*Plantago ovata*) **Myrrh Gum** (*Commiphora myrrha*), **Juniper berries** (*Juniperis communis*), **Squaw vine** (*Mitchella repens*).

Form: Capsule, Sitz bath

PURPOSE: To treat Vaginal Yeast Infection (Vaginitis) and other female problems including cervical, and urinary tract infection.

Other Applications: Unusual bleeding (Menses, Nosebleeds, etc.), Hemorrhoids, Varicose Veins, Difficult Urination, Tonic.

USE: 1. Vaginal yeast infection: 2 caps, 4 times daily. For best results, supplement with 4-6 caps of Garlic per dayand 3-5 caps of the FEVERS & INFECTIONS blend. 1. Urinary Tract Infection: 4-6 caps/day.
2. Cervical Infections: 6 caps/day.
3. To supplement the DIURETIC Blend: 3-4 caps/day.

Contraindications: Persons with known potassium insufficiency should exercise caution and consider using supplemental potassium when using products containing diuretics.

Vaginal infections (vaginitis) may be caused by several means, the most common being yeast (candida albicans); others are bacteria, vitamin B and A deficiencies, intestinal worms and improper hygiene. Every herb in this blend, by some means, has been shown to be effective in reducing symptoms of leukorrhea and related vaginal, cervical and uterine problems. The combined mode of action of these herbs is to soothe inflamed and infected mucous membranes, inhibit discharges, while disinfecting the area in the interest of good health.

GOLDENSEAL ROOT and its major constituent, hydrastine, have been repeatedly proven through global research first, to reduce inflammation of mucous membranes (vaginal and uterine) (**2**), second, to control uterine hemorrhaging (**3**), and third, to destroy harmful bacteria and other germs (**4**). It has been suggested that berberine (a primary constituent of Goldenseal, along with hydrastine) acts on mucosal surfaces by coagulating proteins and thus decreasing the inflammatory congestion (**6**). *(See also INFLUENZA; STOMACH/INTESTINAL; NERVES & GLANDS; FEVERS & INFECTIONS; EYES; HEMORRHOIDS/ASTRINGENT.)*

WITCH HAZEL LEAF possesses a unique kind of astringency whose main locus of action is on the venous system, acting to restore tone, health and vigor throughout that system. It also has a powerful hemostatic property. Hemorrhoids and varicose veins are even benefited by this plant. In fact, almost any sort of minor bleeding such as nosebleed, scratches, etc., can be quickly mended with the application of Witch Hazel tincture or poultice. But the primary usefulness of Witch Hazel leaves is for treating congestive conditions of the uterus, cervix, and vagina, including vaginitis and prolapsus. *(See also HEMORRHOIDS/ASTRINGENT)*

PLANTAIN imparts a necessary soothing mucilage to products designed for internal symptomatic relief of the irritated urinary tract and for external relief of inflamed and painful mucous membranes. The Plantain provides the necessary cooling balm that takes the harsh astringent edge away from the blend. By itself, Plantain has often been used to treat female disorders that are accompanied by fluent discharges. It was used by American Indians, early physicians, and is still used by modern herbalists, to treat hemorrhoids (as well as snakebite, coughs, venereal disease, and countless other ailments). *(See also BONE-FLESH-CARTILAGE; WEIGHT LOSS; RESPIRATORY AILMENTS; CHOLESTEROL REGULATION)*

BUCHU LEAF is a recognized urinary antiseptic (**15**) that acts to eliminate mucous, acid urine and irritation, and is given to combat many forms of inflammation and infection, including cystitis, pyelitis, urethritis, and prostatitis (**16**). *(See also DIURETIC; PROSTATE)*

MYRRH GUM's three great actions are on digestion, infection and vaginitis, the first two of which are discussed in the chapters on STOMACH/INTESTINAL and FEVERS & INFECTIONS. The third effect was observed and recorded several centuries ago in China (**17**). Myrrh gum is antiseptic to mucous membranes, and, curiously, both inhibits oversecretion as well as disinhibits undersecretion of these tissues; thus, it *normalizes mucous membrane activity (13). The anti-infectious nature of Myrrh also plays an active role in this blend. The bacteriostatic and antiseptic properties of the herb have been experimentally verified in both America and China (18-19).* *(See also STOMACH/INTESTINAL; FEVERS & INFECTIONS)*

JUNIPER BERRY has been used in America for a couple of hundred years as a urinary antiseptic, and, by some physicians, to treat vaginitis (**20**). It was recommended for several years in the U.S.P. and N.F. as an emmenagogue (an agent that promotes menstrual flow). Its primary application is as a diuretic. *(See also DIURETIC)*

SQUAW VINE acquired its name because it was popular among many American Indian tribes as an aid to parturition, being used in large quantities during the last few weeks of pregnancy (**15**). The plant was also used extensively to treat several uterine difficulties, including painful menstruation and threat of miscarriage. Some early American physicians used the plant quite successfully (**21**), but it wasn't until 1926 that it gained official recognition and was allowed into the National Formulary. *(See also FEMALE TONIC)*

OTHER NUTRIENTS

VITAMINS
(Daily requirements unless otherwise noted)
Vitamin A *25,000-50,000 I.U.*
Vitamin B Complex—High potency
Vitamin B1 *25-50 mg*
Vitamin B2 *25-50 mg*
Vitamin B6 *25-100 mg*
Vitamin D *400 I.U.*
Vitamin E
Vitamin C *1,000-2,000 mg*
Pantothenic Acid *100 mg*

MINERALS
Zinc
Calcium/Magnesium

MISCELLANEOUS
Nizoral
Digestive enzymes
Essential Fatty Acids
Nystatin
Protein

REFERENCES

1. Chopra, R.N., Dikshit, B.B. & Chowhan, J.S. "Pharmacological action of berberine." **Indian Journal of Medical Research**. 1932, 19(4), 1193-1203.
2. Gibbs, O.S. "On the curious pharmacology of hydrastis." **Federation of American Societies for Experimental Biology Federation Proceedings**. 1947, 6(1), 332.
3. Johnson, C.C., Johnson, G. & Poe, C.F. "Toxicity of alkaloids to certain bacteria. II. Berberine, physostigmine and sanguine." **Acta Pharmacologica et Toxicologica**. 1952, 8(1), 71-78.
4. Sharda, D.C. "Berberine in the treatment of diarrhea of infancy and childhood." **Journal of the Indian Medical Association**, 54(1), 22-24, 1970.
5. Ellingwood, F. **American Materia Medica, Therapeutics and Pharmacognosy**. Eclectic Medical Pubs, Portland, Oregon, 1983.
6. Claus, E.P. **Pharmacognosy**. 4th ed. Lea & Febiger, Philadelphia, 1961.
7. Youngken, H.W. **Textbook of Pharmacognosy**. 5th ed. Blakiston. Philadelphia. 1943.
8. Hartwell, J.L. "Plants used against cancer. A survey." **Lloydia**. 31(2), 71-170, 1968.
9. Kiangsu Institute of Modern Medicine. **Encyclopedia of Chinese Drugs**. 1977. 2 vols. Shanghai Scientific and Technical Publications. Shanghae. People's Republic of China.
10. Majno, G. **The Healing Hand—Man and Wound in the Ancient World**. Harvard University Press, Cambridge, Mass. 1975. 217-218.
11. Gunn, J.C. & Johnson, J.H. **Gunn's Newest Family Physician**. Philadelphia, 1878.
12. Skinner, H.B. **The Family Doctor, Or Guide to Health...** Boston, published for author, 1844.

WEIGHT LOSS

HERBS: **PLANTAIN** (*Plantago ovata*), **Fennel seed** (*Foeniculum vulgare*), **Burdock root** (*Arctium lappa*), **Hawthorn berries** (*Crataegus oxyacantha*), **Kelp** (*Laminaria, Macrocystis, Ascophyllum*), **Bladderwrack** (*Fucus vesiculosus*).

Form: Capsule

PURPOSE: To lose weight safely, naturally and effectively.

Other Applications: Arthritis, gout, edema, high cholesterol levels, psoriasis, appetite suppressant.

USE: 1. While Dieting: 3-4 capsimmediately before each meal with a glass of water.
2. While not Dieting: 2-3 caps/meal.
3. As nutritional supplement during fasts: 4-6 caps/day.

Contraindications: None. If used in conjunction with a diuretic, care should be exercised to avoid serum potassium depletion as may occur when using diuretics.

An herbal supplement to a weight reducing program should supply necessary nutrients, including vitamins, minerals and salts to sustain and nurture vital body systems, including the nerves, glands, skin, blood and organs. In addition, one should expect some help from the product in actually losing pounds. These two purposes are fulfilled by this blend full of Seeds and Seaweed, Berries and Burs. However, if you just sit around, you will not obtain any benefit from the increased metabolic capacity these herbs provide.

NOTE: I have never been satisfied with the use of Chickweed to promote weight loss. No experiment has shown the slightest indication that Chickweed is active in this respect. I have recommended for years that Plantain, an herb whose contribution to weight loss is receiving more scientific substantiation all the time, be used in the place of Chickweed.

PLANTAIN mucilage in the diet dramatically reduces serum cholesterol levels. Plantain before meals causes a definite decrease in triglycerides and beta cholesterol (the bad guys) with a proportional increase of serum levels of alpha cholesterol (the good guy) (**1**). Since deficiency in the latter substance has been implicated in obesity, type II diabetes and atherosclerosis, it is likely that Plantain mucilage provides some protection against those diseases. Plantain in a reducing diet for women has resulted in weight loss substantially greater than that obtained by the diet alone (**2**). Plantain works probably because it satiates the appetite, thereby limiting caloric intake, and because it reduces the absorption of lipids (**3**). *(See also VAGINAL YEAST INFECTION; BONE-FLESH-CARTILAGE; RESPIRATORY PROBLEMS; CHOLESTEROL REGULATION)*

FENNEL was used as a dietary aid as far back as the first century. It is still successfully used today. Fennel does not directly affect weight, rather it has soothing, mildly stimulating properties, that help maintain tone and stasis, that sterilize and stimulate the gastro-intestinal tract, and help reduce griping or cramping (**4**). *(See also DIGESTION)*

BURDOCK ROOT, is included here to help cleanse the blood of toxins during the weight loss regimen. It markedly enhances liver and gall/bile functions (**5-6**). Though the ingestion of Burdock root probably will not lead to weight loss, any good weight loss program should incorporate an herb to strengthen and purify the blood. *(See also DETOXIFY/NURTURE; SKIN PROBLEMS; BONE-FLESH-CARTILAGE; BLOOD PURI/DETOX)*

HAWTHORN BERRY helps to offset the increased demands made on the heart by the condition of being overweight. It also helps recondition and tone up the heart muscle while reducing, especially if the reducing plan includes, as it should, some form of exercise. In that case, it is very important that the heart be able to supply sufficient oxygen to the tissues. Hawthorn berries have been shown to have an oxygen-saving effect on the heart muscle (**7**). Hawthorn also has a very strong vasodilatory action, and it lowers peripheral resistance to blood flow (**8**). After several hours of food abstinence the herb produces a significant decrease in free fatty acids and in lactic acid. (**9**). These findings indicate that Hawthorn has an anabolic, or building up, effect on the metabolic processes, and helps reduce coronary stress induced by overweight and by exercise. *(See also HEART; CHOLESTEROL REGULATION)*

KELP and **BLADDERWRACK** are two of the best weight-reduction plants available. Iodine in Kelp maintains a healthy thyroid, thereby significantly reducing one major cause of obesity. In addition, seaweeds increase the body's ability to burn off fat through exercise (**10**). Stamina is boosted, allowing cells to consume energy more effeciently. Kelp also lowers blood cholesterol levels (**11**).

OTHER NUTRIENTS

VITAMINS
(Daily requirements unless otherwise noted)
Vitamin B-1 *25-100 mg*
Vitamin B-2 *25-100 mg*
Vitamin B-6 *25-100 mg*
Vitamin B-12 *4 mcg*
Vitamin C *500-1,000 mg*
Vitamin E *100-600 I.U.*
Inositol *1,000 mg*
Choline *1,000 mg*

MINERALS
Calcium/Magnesium

MISCELLANEOUS
Lecithin

REFERENCES

1. Frati-Munari, A., Fernandez, H.J.A, Becerril, M., Chavez, N.A., Banales, H.M. "Decrease in serum lipids, glycemia and body weight by plantago in obese and diabetic patients." **Archivos de Investigacion Medica (Mexico)**, 14(3), 259-268, 1983.
2. Enzi, G, Inelmen, E.M. & Crepaldi, G. "Effect of hydrophilic mucilage in the treatment of obese patients." **Pharmatherapeutica**, 2(7), 420-428, 1980.
3. Forman, D.T., Garvin, G.E., Forestner, J.E., & Taylor, C.B. "Increased excretion of fecal bile acids by an oral hydrophillic colloid." **Proceedings of the Society for Experimental and Biological Medicine**, 127, 1060, 1968.
4. Shipochliev, T. "Pharmacological study of several essential oils. I. effect on smooth muscle." **Veterinarno-Meditsinski Nauki**, 5, 63, 1968 (Chem Abstracts 70, 86144e, 1969.
5. Felter, H. W. **The Eclectic Materia Medica, Pharmacology and Therapeutics.** Eclectic Medical Publications, Portland, Oregon, 1983 (first published 1922).
6. Charbrol, E. & Charonnat, R. "Therapeutic agents in bile secretion." **Ann. Med.**, 37, 131-42, 1935.
7. Kandziora, J. "The effects of Crataegus on perfusion disorders of the heart." **Muenchen Medizinische Wochenschrift**, 111(6), 295-298, 1969.
8. Kovach, A.G.B., Foedl, M. & Fedina, L. "Effects of extract obtained from Crataegus oxyacantha on Coronary blood flow in dogs." **Arzneimittelforschungen**, 9(6), 378-379, 1959.
9. Hammerl, H., Kranzl, C., Pichler, O., & Studlar, M. "Clinical and experimental investigations on metabolism using an extract of Crataegus." **Arztliche Forschung**, 21(7), 261-264, 1967.
10. Johnston, H.W. "Composition of edible seaweeds." **Proceedings of the Seventh International Seaweed Symposium**. Wiley and Sons, New York, 1972, pp. 429-435.
11. Kimura, A. & Kuramoto, M. "Influences of seaweeds of metabolism of cholesterol and anticoagulant actions of seaweed." **Tokushima Journal of Experimental Medicine**, 21, 79-88, 1974.

TONIC—WHOLE BODY

HERBS: SARSAPARILLA root (*Smilax officinalis*), **Siberian** GINSENG (*Eleutherococcus senticosus*), **Fo-Ti** (*Polygonum multiflorum, ho-shou-wu*), **Gotu Kola** (*Hydrocotyle asiatica*), **Saw Palmetto berries** (*Serenoa repens-sabal*) **Licorice root** (*Glycyrrhiza glabra*), **Kelp** (*Laminaria, Macrocystis, Ascophyllum*), **Stillingia** (*Stillingia sylvatica*), **Alfalfa** (*Medicago sativa*), & **Cayenne** (*Capsicum annum*).

Form: Capsule.

PURPOSE: To supplement all other blends in this manual; to use daily as a regular dietary supplement; to increase vitality.

Other Applications: Longevity.

USE: 2-12 caps/day as desired. Generally, use more during periods of convalescence, poor health and high stress.

Contraindications: None.

This blend is *the* ultimate tonic. The blend contains the true heavy-weights of the herbal kingdom. This blend is for those who are really serious about wholistic health, those who cherish the daily rejuvenation of the body's vital substances, the inexorable growth of stamina, strength and resistance to disease. Use it with impunity. There is not a gland, nerve, muscle, vein, artery, organ, or bone in the body that will not experience significant benefits. The longer you maintain daily usage, the greater those benefits will be.

SARSAPARILLA belongs to a large family of related *Smilax* species, the members of which are used in countries around the world for fairly similar purposes. But nowhere except in the United States has this herb attained the status of tonic. Americans learned about the uses of Sarsaparilla from the Indians. The plant is used for coughs, hypertension, pleurisy, wounds, sore eyes, burns, as a diuretic and alterative, and most importantly as a general tonic. *(See also INFERTILITY, ARTHRITIS, BLOOD PURIFIER/DETOXIFIER, DETOXIFY/NURTURE.)*

SIBERIAN GINSENG is the ultimate example of man's almost mystical interaction with nature. Because of its antiquity and shape, Ginseng plays the central role in a good deal of Chinese mythology, medicine, commerce and trade. For Western man, the economic value of Ginseng outweighed its medicinal value until the past 15 years or so, during which time research on the plant has grown explosively, and has tended to verify and extend the medicinal claims. Ginseng has been found to: stimulate the central nervous system in small amounts and depress the Central Nervous System in large doses; protect the body and nervous system from stress; stimulate and increase metabolic function; increase physical and mental efficiency; lower blood pressure and glucose levels when high, and raise them when low; increase gastrointestinal movement and tone; increase iron metabolism; and cause changes in nucleic acid (RNA) biosynthesis. *(See also INFERTILITY, FATIGUE, WHOLE BODY TONIC, MENTAL ALERTNESS/SENILITY, BLOOD SUGAR.)*

FO-TI has been found to reduce hypertension, blood cholesterol levels and the incidence of coronary heart disease among individuals prone to these conditions. (**1**). In Chinese materia medica Fo-Ti is used for neurasthenia, insomnia, sweating, dizziness, elevated serum cholesterol, coronary disease, weakness, pain, backache, and tuberculous adenopathy (**2**). These uses conform to the traditional Chinese medical view that Fo-Ti has anti-toxic, anti-swelling and tranquilizing properties (**3**).

GOTU KOLA is a traditional Asian blood purifier, tonic and diuretic. It is commonly used for diseases of the skin, blood and nervous system. Gotu Kola contains asiaticoside which is being used in the Far East to treat leprosy and tuberculosis. Unlike the pronounced, quick acting anti-fatigue property of Capsicum (which is also in this blend) a *combination* of Ginseng and Gotu Kola have been found to gradually increase the overal energy or activity levels (**4-5**). Gotu Kola contains no caffeine at all. Kola nut contains caffeine. They are not the same plant, or even remotely related. *(See also FATIGUE, MENTAL ALERTNESS/SENILITY, BLOOD SUGAR.)*

SAW PALMETTO BERRIES See TONIC—NERVE & GLAND for tonic information. F r particulars, see INFERTILITY, RESPIRATORY AILMENTS, DIABETES, FEMALE TONIC, PROSTATE, NERVES & GLANDS, THYROID, and DIGESTION.

LICORICE ROOT, for good reasons, is contained in many of the blends recommended in this book. Besides possessing numerous specific medicinal properties, it modulates and strengthens the activity of other herbs. In both Western and Eastern medicine Licorice root plays a central role, and is used in both cultures for almost exactly the same conditions. Licorice root's status as a tonic is undoubtedly due to the cumulative effect of all its medicinal properties. The herb can be used with impunity. *(See also INFERTILITY, ARTHRITIS, RESPIRATORY AILMENTS, SKIN, FEMALE TONIC, BLOOD PURI/DETOX, LAXATIVE, LIVER DISORDERS, STOMACH/INTESTINAL, DETOXIFY/NURTURE, FEVERS & INFECTIONS, NAUSEA, and BLOOD SUGAR.)*

KELP See TONIC—NERVE & GLAND for information on its tonic activity. For details on specific activity see many other blends in this manual, but especially THYROID, ARTHRITIS, HEART, HIGH BLOOD PRESSURE, CIRCULATION, ENVIRONMENTAL POLLUTION, DETOXIFY/NURTURE, FEVERS & INFECTIONS, and WEIGHT LOSS.

STILLINGIA is discussed under DETOXIFIER/NUTRITIONAL SUPPLEMENT.

ALFALFA is an appetite stimulant and vitality augmenter. The idea of humans eating something generally grown for animals has never really caught on in a big way with the general public, yet is completely accepted by persons interested in natural health. As a spring tonic, Alfalfa has no equal. It is one the best sources for protein. In addition, it is very high in vitamins A, D, E, B-6, and K, calcium, magnesium, chlorophyll, phosphorous, iron, potassium, trace minerals and several digestive enzymes. The chapter on ARTHRITIS discusses Alfalfa's role further. *(See also ENVIRONMENTAL POLLUTION.)*

CAYENNE See TONIC—NERVE & GLAND for information on its tonic value. *(See also CIRCULATION; HIGH BLOOD PRESSURE; FATIGUE; INFLUENZA; BLOOD PURIFICATION/DETOXIFICATION)*

OTHER NUTRIENTS

VITAMINS
(Daily requirements unless otherwise noted)
Vitamin A *25,000 I.U.*
Vitamin B Complex
Vitamin B1 *25 mg*
Vitamin B2 *25 mg*
Vitamin B6 *25 mg*
Vitamin B12 *25 mcg*
Vitamin C *500 mg*
Vitamin D *400 I.U.*
Vitamin E *200 I.U.*
Biotin *150 mcg*
Niacinamide *50 mg*
PABA *30 mg*
Pantothenic Acid *100 mg*
Choline *1,000 mg*
Inositol *1,000 mg*
Bioflavonoids *100 mg*
Folic Acid *400 mcg*

MINERALS
Calcium/Magnesium
Zinc
Selenium
Phosphorous
Manganese
Iron
Copper
Iodine
Chromium

MISCELLANEOUS
GLA
Essential Fatty Acid
Lecithin
Protein
Brewer's Yeast
Yogurt
Wheat Germ
HCl

REFERENCES

1. Zhuo, D. "Preventive geriatrics: an overview from traditional chinese medicine." **American Journal of Chinese Medicine**, 10(1-4), 32-39, 1982.
2. Cheung, S.C. & Li, N.H. (eds) "Polygonum multiflorum Thumb." In **Chinese Medicinal Herbs of Hong Kong**, 1980.
3. Kam, J.K. "Mutagenic activity of Ho Shao Wu (Polygonum multiflorum Thumb)". **American Journal of Chinese Medicine**, 9(3), 213-215, 1981.
4. Mowrey, D.B. "Capsicum, Ginseng and Gotu Kola in combination." **The Herbalist**, Premier issue, 22-28, 1975.
5. Mowrey, D.B. "The effects of Capsicum, Gotu Kola and Ginseng on activity: further evidence." **The Herbalist**, 1(1), 51-54, 1976.

INDEX